Juicing for Kidney Health.

A Guide to Supporting Renal Function with Fresh Juice"

Disa Sophie

Juicing for Kidney Health

Juicing for Kidney Health

Table of contents.

Contents

Juicing for Kidney Health

Juicing for Kidney Health

Juicing for Kidney Health

Juicing for Kidney Health

Juicing for Kidney Health

Juicing for Kidney Health

Juicing for Kidney Health

Juicing for Kidney Health

INTRODUCTION TO JUICING FOR KIDNEY HEALTH

Victoria is a 35-year-old mother of two. She was always on the go, working long hours as a nurse and taking care of her family. Despite her hectic schedule, she made an effort to eat a nutritious diet and stay active. She had no idea she had any health problems until she went in for a routine check-up and was told she had early-stage chronic kidney disease (CKD).

Victoria was stunned and couldn't comprehend how this could have happened to her. She had no visible symptoms and appeared to be totally healthy. Her doctor stated that CKD is a quiet and progressive ailment with little symptoms in the early stages. He advised her to take care of her kidneys in order to prevent the condition from progressing.

She took the news to heart and made some lifestyle modifications. She began drinking more water and eating a diet low in salt, sugar, and fat. She also made an effort to manage her stress and keep physically active. She also began monitoring her blood pressure and blood sugar levels, as well as taking medications as advised to control her underlying medical issues.

Her doctor was amazed by her dedication to her health and how she had changed her lifestyle. He told her that her kidney function had improved and that she was on the right track to preventing the advancement of her condition. Victoria felt pleased with herself and motivated to keep up her good habits.

Victoria's experience emphasizes the necessity of understanding the role of the kidneys in our bodies and taking care of our health. She discovered that early detection and preventative interventions can go a long way toward preserving kidney function and delaying the progression of renal disease. She was able to improve her general well-being and protect her health for years to come by making informed health decisions and taking care of her kidneys.

The process of juicing involves removing the juice from fruits and vegetables. It's an excellent method to get a lot of vitamins, minerals, and antioxidants in one meal. Juicing can be very helpful for kidney patients because it helps enhance kidney function and stop further damage.

Juicing for Kidney Health

Filtering waste materials and extra fluid from the circulation is a critical function of the kidneys. Renal damage can develop over time as a result of toxic drug exposure and poor eating habits, which can result in kidney disease and kidney failure, among other health issues.

Juicing gives the body the nutrients it needs to function properly, which can help preserve kidney health. Fresh juices include a high concentration of vitamins, minerals, and antioxidants that can enhance general health and lower the risk of kidney injury.

The following are some of the top fruits and vegetables for kidney health:

Cranberries: By preventing bacteria from adhering to the urinary tract, cranberries can lower the incidence of urinary tract infections.

Cucumbers: Due to their high water and electrolyte content, cucumbers can help the body remove harmful toxins and lower the risk of kidney injury.

Beets: Beets have a lot of nitrates, which can help the kidneys get more oxygen and blood flow.

Leafy greens: Leafy greens are rich in vitamins and minerals, including vitamins A and C, iron, and potassium. Examples of leafy greens include spinach and kale.

Apples: Pectin, which can help lower cholesterol and prevent kidney damage, is a good source of nutrition in apples.

It is crucial to remember that while juicing might be useful for preserving kidney function, a balanced diet should always come first. Lean proteins, whole grains, and a variety of fruits and vegetables should still be consumed to preserve general health and stop additional kidney injury.

In conclusion, by supplying the body with vital vitamins, minerals, and antioxidants, juicing can be a terrific approach to enhancing kidney health. You can lessen the risk of kidney damage and maintain general health by adding a range of healthful fruits and vegetables to your juice.

Juicing for Kidney Health

CHAPTER 1

Understanding the Importance of Kidney Function.

The human body is a sophisticated and complicated system, with numerous organs interacting harmoniously to sustain general health. In this system, the kidneys are essential because they filter wastes and extra fluids from the blood and expel them from the body in the form of urine. Additionally, the kidneys control the electrolyte balance, generate the hormones that control blood pressure and red blood cell formation, and encourage the production of more red blood cells in the bone marrow.

Understanding the significance of renal function is essential since kidney disease is a quiet, progressive disorder that, if unchecked, can cause a variety of health issues. Millions of people throughout the world suffer from chronic kidney disease (CKD), which is defined by a long-term deterioration in kidney function. Early CKD is difficult to detect and diagnose since it frequently has no obvious symptoms. Anemia, nerve damage, fluid retention, and heart disease are just a few of the signs and problems that can develop as the condition worsens.

For overall health, it's crucial to maintain healthy kidney function, and there are several ways to do this. Maintaining a balanced diet low in salt, sugar, and animal protein as well as staying hydrated will support kidney health. Additionally, it's critical to manage any underlying medical disorders like high blood pressure, diabetes, or heart disease because these can put stress on the kidneys and hasten the development of CKD.

Kidneys play a vital role in filtering waste products.

The kidneys are intricate and important organs that serve the body in a number of key ways. Filtering waste materials and extra fluid from the circulation and eliminating them through urine is one of the kidneys' most crucial jobs. This procedure is necessary for preserving overall health and preventing the buildup of toxic substances in the body.

The nephrons in the kidneys are little organs that filter the blood that is continuously supplied to them. Wastes, poisons, and extra fluid are expelled as urine after being separated from the blood within each nephron and delivered to the renal pelvis. The filtered blood is subsequently sent

Juicing for Kidney Health

back into the system. To keep the body free of waste and poisons, this process is carried out continually, around the clock.

The health of the kidneys and other organs in the body can be learned from the information contained in urine, which is more than just a waste product. Various health issues, such as renal disease, dehydration, or urinary tract infections, might be indicated by changes in the color, odor, or volume of urine, for instance.

The balance of electrolytes in the body is regulated by the kidneys, which also filter waste materials and extra fluid. Minerals called electrolytes, such as sodium, potassium, and calcium, are crucial for healthy body operations. By reabsorbing the necessary electrolytes and excreting the rest, the kidneys control the blood's electrolyte levels. As a result, significant health issues, including high blood pressure and heart disease, are avoided, and the right electrolyte balance is maintained.

The kidneys are crucial in filtering wastes and extra fluids from the blood and excreting them in the form of urine. This procedure is necessary for preserving overall health and preventing the buildup of toxic substances in the body. A healthy lifestyle can help maintain kidney function and stave off the onset of renal disease. Regular kidney function monitoring is one way to do this.

Kidneys regulate the balance of electrolytes and produce hormones that regulate blood pressure.

The kidneys are crucial for filtering waste and extra fluid, but they are also essential for maintaining the proper balance of electrolytes and creating hormones that control a number of body processes.

Minerals called electrolytes, such as sodium, potassium, and calcium, are crucial for healthy body operations. The kidneys assist in controlling the amount of electrolytes in the blood by reabsorbing the ones that are required and excreting the remainder in urine. As a result, significant health issues, including high blood pressure, heart disease, and muscular cramps, are avoided, and the right electrolyte balance is maintained.

Juicing for Kidney Health

The kidneys produce hormones that are crucial in controlling a variety of body activities in addition to electrolyte balance. Erythropoietin, a hormone generated by the kidneys, encourages the bone marrow to make more red blood cells. This assists in preserving the body's healthy red blood cell balance and preventing anemia.

Renin, another hormone that the kidneys generate and which controls blood pressure, instructs the body to create the hormone angiotensin II, which tightens blood vessels and raises blood pressure. This aids in controlling blood pressure and makes sure that the body's organs and tissues receive adequate amounts of oxygen and nutrients.

Calcitriol, another hormone made by the kidneys, aids in controlling the body's calcium and phosphorus levels. This promotes strong bones and teeth and guards against significant health issues like osteoporosis.

The generation of hormones that control numerous biological activities, such as blood pressure and the creation of red blood cells, as well as the balancing of electrolytes, are crucial tasks of the kidneys. For general health, maintaining strong kidney function is crucial. There are several ways to do this, including by drinking plenty of water, eating a balanced diet, and controlling underlying medical issues. Regular renal function monitoring and health decision-making can help maintain kidney function and halt the emergence of major health issues.

Chronic Kidney Disease (CKD) is a silent and progressive condition.

Chronic Kidney Disease (CKD) is a silent and progressive disease that affects millions of people around the world. It is a chronic disorder in which the kidneys gradually lose function over time, resulting in a variety of major health issues and, finally, end-stage renal disease (ESRD).

Because symptoms may not develop until the disease is advanced, CKD is sometimes referred to as a "silent" disorder. There may be no symptoms in the early stages, but as the disease progresses, symptoms may include weariness, loss of appetite, swelling in the legs and ankles, and a decrease in urine production.

Because it worsens over time, CKD is considered a progressive condition, and there is presently no cure. The kidneys lose their ability to adequately filter waste products and excess fluid from

Juicing for Kidney Health

the circulation as the disease advances, resulting in a buildup of toxins and waste products in the body. This can lead to a variety of major health issues, such as anemia, nerve damage, bone disease, and cardiovascular disease.

Diabetes, high blood pressure, and autoimmune illnesses are some of the conditions that can cause CKD. A family history of renal disease, smoking, obesity, and being older than 60 are all risk factors for having CKD.

Early detection and treatment of CKD are critical for decreasing disease development and preventing significant health issues. Regular renal function testing, management of underlying medical illnesses, a nutritious diet, and regular exercise can all help to delay the progression of CKD and prevent its significant health consequences. In advanced stages of the disease, dialysis or kidney transplantation may be alternatives.

To summarize, chronic kidney disease (CKD) is a silent and progressive disease that affects millions of individuals worldwide. It is a chronic disorder in which the kidneys gradually lose function over time, resulting in a variety of major health issues and, finally, end-stage renal disease (ESRD). Early detection and treatment of CKD are critical for decreasing disease development and preventing significant health issues.

Early stages of CKD often have no noticeable symptoms.

The early stages of chronic kidney disease (CKD) sometimes have no apparent symptoms, making it difficult to detect and diagnose. This is why CKD is often referred to as a "silent" disease. Many people may have the problem for years without realizing it and may not seek medical assistance until the sickness is severe.

The kidneys are highly resilient organs that can compensate for reduced function in the early stages of CKD. As a result, even if a large amount of kidney function is lost, there may be no obvious symptoms. Only after a significant percentage of kidney function has been lost may symptoms such as weariness, loss of appetite, swelling in the legs and ankles, and a decrease in urine production develop.

Juicing for Kidney Health

The lack of visible symptoms in the early stages of CKD makes it difficult for individuals to recognize the ailment and seek medical assistance. It also makes it more difficult for healthcare personnel to recognize and diagnose the problem in its early stages, as they may not suspect the presence of kidney disease based only on symptoms.

Early detection and diagnosis of CKD are critical because the earlier the disease is diagnosed, the more successful treatment can be in slowing disease development and averting significant health consequences. Regular monitoring of kidney function via blood and urine testing can help diagnose the disease in its early stages and allow for early treatment.

The early stages of chronic kidney disease (CKD) sometimes have no apparent symptoms, making it difficult to detect and diagnose. The lack of apparent symptoms in the early stages of the disease makes it difficult for individuals to recognize they have the condition and seek medical attention, as well as for healthcare providers to detect and diagnose the disease. Regular monitoring of renal function is critical for early detection and efficient treatment of CKD.

Progressive CKD can lead to a host of symptoms and complications.

Chronic Kidney Disease (CKD) is a chronic disorder that worsens over time and can cause a variety of symptoms and problems. As the condition advances, the kidneys lose their ability to properly filter waste products and excess fluid from the blood, resulting in a buildup of toxins and waste products in the body. This can result in a variety of major health issues, including anemia, nerve damage, fluid retention, and heart disease.

Anemia is a typical consequence of CKD that happens when the kidneys are unable to produce enough erythropoietin, a hormone that encourages the creation of red blood cells. As a result, there may not be enough red blood cells to deliver oxygen throughout the body, resulting in weariness and weakness.

Nerve damage, or neuropathy, can also occur as a result of CKD. This can result in a variety of symptoms, including tingling, numbness, and pain in the extremities. Nerve injury can be caused by a buildup of waste products in the bloodstream as well as inadequate blood flow caused by a decline in kidney function.

Juicing for Kidney Health

Fluid retention is another common consequence of CKD that arises when the kidneys are unable to properly eliminate excess fluid from the body. This might cause edema and shortness of breath, especially while resting.

Heart disease is another major consequence of CKD. This can happen because a buildup of waste products and fluid in the body can generate high blood pressure, which can damage the blood vessels and heart. This can increase the risk of a heart attack, stroke, and other cardiovascular disorders.

Chronic Kidney Disease (CKD) is a degenerative condition that can cause a variety of symptoms and problems, including anemia, nerve damage, fluid retention, and heart disease. As the condition advances, the kidneys lose their capacity to adequately filter waste products and excess fluid from the blood, resulting in a buildup of toxins and waste products in the body that can cause major health concerns. Regular monitoring of renal function and early treatment of underlying medical issues can help delay the progression of CKD and prevent significant health complications.

Maintaining good kidney function is essential for overall health.

Good kidney function is critical for general health and well-being. The kidneys are responsible for filtering waste products and excess fluids from the blood and excreting them as urine. When the kidneys are working properly, they help maintain electrolyte balance, regulate blood pressure, and create hormones that control red blood cell development.

Individuals can make many efforts to preserve normal kidney function and prevent the development of chronic kidney disease (CKD). These are some examples:

Hydration: Drinking plenty of water and other fluids can aid in the correct functioning of the kidneys. Staying hydrated can help prevent kidney stones and lower the risk of kidney injury.

A healthy diet that is high in fruits, vegetables, and whole grains and low in salt, sugar, and fat can help keep kidney function in check. A healthy diet can also help control blood pressure and prevent the development of CKD.

Juicing for Kidney Health

Managing Substantial Medical Conditions: Substantial medical conditions such as diabetes and high blood pressure can raise the risk of kidney injury and should be addressed by lifestyle changes and medical treatment. Regular blood sugar and blood pressure monitoring, as well as taking medications as directed, can help avoid the progression of these disorders and safeguard renal function.

Avoiding Harmful Substances: Substance misuse, such as heavy alcohol intake, smoking, and drug use, can harm the kidneys significantly. Avoiding these toxic chemicals can aid in the maintenance of excellent renal function and the prevention of the development of CKD.

Regular Check-Ups: Visiting a healthcare professional on a regular basis will help monitor kidney function and discover any early signs of renal disease. Regular monitoring of kidney function using blood and urine tests can aid in the early detection of CKD and allow for early therapy.

Good kidney function is critical for general health and well-being. Simple efforts like hydration, a nutritious diet, controlling underlying medical issues, avoiding hazardous substances, and scheduling frequent check-ups with a healthcare practitioner can help preserve excellent kidney function and prevent the development of chronic kidney disease (CKD). Taking care of one's kidneys is a crucial part of staying healthy and avoiding significant health concerns.

Regular check-ups with a healthcare provider.

Regular medical check-ups, a healthy lifestyle, and addressing underlying medical issues are all important steps in preserving kidney function and preventing the progression of renal disease.

Regular Check-Ups: Regular check-ups with a healthcare professional can help monitor kidney function and detect any early signs of renal disease. Regular blood and urine tests to evaluate kidney function can help diagnose kidney disease in its early stages and allow for early treatment. This can help retain kidney function and slow the course of renal disease.

Healthy Lifestyle Choices: Making nutritious lifestyle choices, such as eating healthy foods, staying hydrated, and avoiding dangerous substances, can help retain kidney function and prevent the advancement of renal disease. A diet high in fruits, vegetables, and whole grains and

Juicing for Kidney Health

low in salt, sugar, and fat can help maintain healthy kidney function. Staying hydrated can help avoid the production of kidney stones and lower the risk of kidney injury. Substance misuse, such as heavy alcohol drinking, smoking, and drug use, can cause considerable kidney damage and should be avoided.

Managing Underlying Medical Disorders: Managing underlying medical conditions such as diabetes and high blood pressure can help preserve kidney function and prevent the advancement of kidney disease. Regular blood sugar and blood pressure monitoring, as well as taking medications as prescribed, can help avoid the progression of these disorders and safeguard renal function.

In conclusion, maintaining kidney function is critical for general health and well-being. Regular check-ups with a healthcare professional, adopting a healthy lifestyle, and controlling underlying medical issues can all assist in retaining kidney function and preventing the advancement of renal disease. Taking care of the kidneys is a crucial part of staying healthy and avoiding significant health problems.

Taking care of our kidneys is an important part of maintaining overall health and wellness.

Taking care of our kidneys is a vital element of overall health and fitness. Our kidneys perform an important role in filtering waste products and excess fluids from the circulation and excreting them in the form of urine. They also maintain electrolyte balance and create hormones that regulate blood pressure and red blood cell synthesis. Understanding their function in our bodies can help us make more informed health decisions.

Kidneys are critical organs that perform numerous important activities in our bodies. They filter waste items and excess fluids from the circulation and expel them in the form of urine. They help maintain the equilibrium of electrolytes such as sodium, potassium, and calcium, which are required for the normal functioning of our cells and tissues. They also generate hormones that regulate blood pressure and increase the creation of red blood cells.

Juicing for Kidney Health

Understanding the Role of the Kidneys: Understanding the role of the kidneys in our bodies might help us make more educated health decisions. To maintain kidney function, for example, we can stay hydrated and eat a balanced diet low in salt, sugar, and fat. We can also monitor our blood pressure and blood sugar levels and take drugs as prescribed to control underlying medical problems that can impair kidney function, such as diabetes and high blood pressure.

The Importance of Prevention: Chronic Kidney Disease (CKD) is a silent and degenerative disorder that affects millions of individuals worldwide. Early stages of CKD frequently have no apparent symptoms, making it difficult to detect and diagnose. Progressive CKD can cause a variety of symptoms and problems, including anemia, nerve damage, fluid retention, and heart disease. Maintaining healthy kidney function and limiting the advancement of renal disease is thus critical for overall health and well-being.

Healthy Lifestyle Choices: Making healthy lifestyle choices can help retain kidney function and reduce the advancement of renal disease. Eating a well-balanced diet high in fruits, vegetables, and whole grains and low in salt, sugar, and fat will help maintain optimal kidney function. Staying hydrated can help avoid the production of kidney stones and lower the risk of kidney injury. Substance misuse, such as heavy alcohol drinking, smoking, and drug use, can cause considerable kidney damage and should be avoided.

In summary, taking care of our kidneys is a crucial element of overall health and wellness. Understanding their role in our bodies and making informed health decisions can help us preserve kidney function and prevent the advancement of renal disease. Regular check-ups with a healthcare practitioner, adopting a healthy lifestyle, and addressing underlying medical disorders can all assist to retain kidney function and protect our health for years to come.

It is critical to comprehend the significance of renal function because the kidneys are essential for preserving general health and wellness. Regular medical checkups, leading a healthy lifestyle, and taking care of underlying medical issues can all help maintain kidney function and stop the progression of renal disease.

In conclusion, the kidneys are an important organ in the human body because they filter waste materials, regulate the electrolyte balance, and produce hormones that are necessary for overall health and wellness. As chronic kidney disease is a widespread and frequently silent ailment that

Juicing for Kidney Health

can cause a variety of health issues if left untreated, it is imperative to comprehend the significance of renal function.

There are numerous ways to maintain healthy kidney function, which is crucial for overall health. Drinking enough water and following a balanced diet low in salt, sugar, and animal protein can support the maintenance of healthy kidney function. Additionally, it's crucial to manage any underlying medical disorders like high blood pressure, diabetes, or heart disease because these can strain the kidneys and hasten the advancement of chronic kidney disease.

Maintaining kidney function and halting the progression of renal disease can be achieved through routine check-ups with a healthcare professional, adopting a healthy lifestyle, and controlling underlying medical issues. Kidney illness can be treated early on to improve quality of life and prevent the onset of significant health issues.

The significance of renal health cannot be overemphasized. Taking care of our kidneys is crucial to maintaining general health and wellness, and being aware of the function of our kidneys in the body can help us make wise decisions regarding our health.

Juicing for Kidney Health

CHAPTER 2

Understanding Kidney Health Issues and How Juicing Can Help

Timmy is a middle-aged man who has always been health-conscious. He had always been into fitness and eating well, but he had been feeling tired and run down recently. He went to the doctor and was astonished to learn that he had kidney difficulties. His doctor informed him that he had early-stage chronic kidney disease (CKD) and that he needed to take care of his kidneys to prevent the disease from progressing.

He was determined to find a remedy that would help him improve his kidney health. He began investigating natural cures and came across information on juicing. He discovered that juicing could assist and promote kidney function by giving the kidneys critical vitamins, minerals, and antioxidants that they require to operate effectively.

Timmy began juicing as part of his daily regimen, making sure to include a variety of fruits and vegetables. He drank fresh juices packed with vegetables like beets, carrots, apples, and ginger, which are known to help with kidney function. He also reduced his intake of processed meals and increased his water intake to aid in the removal of waste and poisons from his body.

He observed a huge difference in his energy levels and overall health after just a few weeks of juicing. His doctor was likewise delighted with his development and informed him that his kidney function had improved. Timmy was so pleased with the results that he decided to make juicing a permanent part of his healthy lifestyle.

His tale emphasizes the importance of knowing renal health issues and how simple changes to our food and lifestyle may help improve our health. He discovered that juicing can help sustain kidney function and slow the advancement of renal disease. He was able to enhance his kidney function and preserve his general well-being by taking charge of his health and adopting intelligent dietary choices.

The kidneys are vital to our body's functioning and general wellness. They are in charge of filtering waste products and surplus fluids from the blood, balancing electrolytes, and creating

Juicing for Kidney Health

hormones that regulate blood pressure and red blood cell development. When the kidneys do not work properly, it can cause a variety of health problems, including chronic renal disease (CKD).

CKD is a silent and progressive disease that affects millions of individuals worldwide. Early stages of CKD frequently have no apparent symptoms, making it difficult to detect and diagnose. Progressive CKD can cause a slew of symptoms and consequences over time.

Maintaining strong kidney function is critical for general health and can be accomplished through water, a nutritious diet, and the management of underlying medical disorders. Juicing is one such diet that has gained popularity in recent years. Juicing is the process of extracting the juice from fresh fruits and vegetables and drinking it to acquire their nutrients.

Juicing can assist in promoting kidney health by supplying vital vitamins, minerals, and antioxidants that the kidneys require to operate effectively. We may help our kidneys and enhance our overall health and wellness by integrating fresh, nutrient-rich juices into our diet.

In this chapter, we will look at the importance of recognizing kidney health issues and how juicing can help support kidney function and prevent the advancement of kidney disease. We will go through the importance of the kidneys in our bodies, the causes and symptoms of CKD, and the benefits of juicing for kidney health.

Importance of understanding kidney health issues

Understanding the significance of kidney health is critical for maintaining overall health and preventing the development of major health problems. The kidneys are two small, bean-shaped organs placed near the center of the back, slightly below the ribcage. They are essential in filtering waste items and excess fluids from the circulation and excreting them in the form of urine.

The kidneys also manage the balance of electrolytes in the body, which include minerals such as sodium, potassium, and calcium that are required for many of the body's processes. They also generate hormones that regulate blood pressure and increase the creation of red blood cells.

Juicing for Kidney Health

When the kidneys do not work properly, it can lead to a variety of health problems, including chronic renal disease (CKD). CKD is a silent and progressive disease that affects millions of individuals worldwide. One in every 10 people is expected to have CKD, and the number is growing as the global population ages.

Early stages of CKD frequently have no apparent symptoms, making it difficult to detect and diagnose. Fatigue, muscular cramps, joint discomfort, swelling, and difficulty concentrating are some of the symptoms that might arise in the later stages of CKD. Progressive CKD can cause a variety of symptoms and problems, including anemia, nerve damage, fluid retention, and heart disease.

In addition to these symptoms and problems, CKD can increase the chance of developing additional significant health diseases such as cardiovascular disease and renal failure. Kidney failure, commonly known as end-stage renal disease (ESRD), is a serious and potentially fatal condition that necessitates dialysis or a kidney transplant.

For these reasons, it is critical to recognize the significance of renal health and to make efforts to preserve proper kidney function. This includes regular check-ups with a healthcare practitioner, adopting a healthy lifestyle, and controlling underlying medical issues. We may improve our overall health and wellness by knowing the importance of renal health and making efforts to support our kidneys.

The causes and symptoms of CKD.

Chronic Kidney Disease (CKD) is a long-term illness in which the kidneys gradually lose their ability to function correctly. This can cause a variety of major health problems, including renal failure, which requires dialysis or a kidney transplant to survive.

There are various causes of CKD, including:

Diabetes: High blood sugar levels can damage the blood vessels in the kidneys, resulting in CKD.

High blood pressure can damage the blood vessels in the kidneys and contribute to CKD.

Juicing for Kidney Health

Glomerulonephritis is a group of kidney illnesses that cause inflammation and damage to the microscopic filters in the kidneys known as glomeruli.

Polycystic Kidney Disease: This is a hereditary disorder that causes fluid-filled cysts to grow in the kidneys, causing damage and eventually the destruction of normal kidney tissue.

Kidney Stones: Kidney stones can cause obstructions in the urinary tract, which can lead to kidney damage and CKD.

Nephrotic Syndrome: This is a set of renal illnesses that produce excessive protein loss in the urine, which can lead to kidney damage and CKD.

Chronic or repeated kidney infections can cause kidney damage over time, leading to CKD.

CKD frequently has no visible symptoms in its early stages, making it difficult to detect and diagnose. However, as the condition advances, the following symptoms may appear:

Fatigue and weakness

Nausea and loss of appetite

Leg, ankle, and foot swelling

Skin that is dry and itchy

Poor concentration and difficulties thinking

Muscle spasms at night

Insomnia and other sleep issues

Changes in urine output and frequency

Sexual dysfunction

It is critical to seek medical attention if you encounter any of these symptoms, as early detection and treatment of CKD can help limit the disease's progression and prevent major health issues. Additionally, regular check-ups with a healthcare professional and addressing underlying medical disorders such as high blood pressure and diabetes can help preserve kidney function and prevent the advancement of renal disease.

Juicing for Kidney Health

Juicing can be an effective strategy to promote kidney function and enhance overall health. Juicing is the process of extracting the juice from fruits and vegetables and drinking it. This procedure offers the body a concentrated concentration of nutrients, such as vitamins, minerals, antioxidants, and phytochemicals, which can help support the kidneys and prevent the development of renal disease.

It can also assist in promoting kidney function by providing the body with critical vitamins and minerals such as vitamin C, potassium, and magnesium. These nutrients are essential for keeping healthy kidneys and can help avoid the progression of renal disease. For example, potassium regulates fluid balance in the body and can help avoid fluid buildup, which is a common indication of kidney illness.

Juicing, in addition to providing important nutrients to the body, can help to maintain kidney function by lowering the amount of toxic chemicals in the body. A diet high in processed foods and sugar can raise waste products and toxins in the body, putting strain on the kidneys and leading to renal disease. Juicing can help remove these toxic compounds from the body and minimize the stress on the kidneys.

Finally, it can assist in improving kidney function by giving the body antioxidants, which are molecules that protect cells from injury. Antioxidants can help avoid oxidative stress and inflammation, both of which are risk factors for kidney disease. We can help support the kidneys and prevent the advancement of renal disease by consuming an antioxidant-rich diet, such as juicing.

To summarize, juicing can be an excellent strategy to promote kidney function and enhance overall health. It can help prevent the advancement of renal disease and promote kidney function by supplying important nutrients, decreasing toxic chemicals, and providing antioxidants. However, before beginning a juicing plan, consult with a healthcare physician because some fruits and vegetables can mix with certain drugs and have a harmful impact on the kidneys.

Juicing for Kidney Health

It prevents the progression of kidney disease.

Juicing can help prevent the progression of kidney disease by providing the body with needed nutrients and lowering toxic compound levels. A diet high in fruits and vegetables, such as juicing, can help promote kidney function and avoid the development of renal disease.

It can help prevent kidney disease by lowering oxidative stress and inflammation. These are common risk factors for kidney disease, and adopting an antioxidant-rich diet, such as through juicing, can help protect the kidneys from damage. Antioxidants are molecules that protect cells from harm and aid in the prevention of oxidative stress and inflammation, both of which can contribute to the progression of kidney disease.

Juicing also help prevent kidney disease by lowering waste and toxin levels in the body. A diet high in processed foods and sugar can raise waste products and toxins in the body, putting strain on the kidneys and leading to renal disease. It can help remove these toxic compounds from the body and minimize the stress on the kidneys.

Furthermore, it helps avoid kidney disease by maintaining a healthy blood pressure. Renin, a hormone produced by the kidneys, aids in the regulation of blood pressure. Juicing has been demonstrated to help lower blood pressure and minimize the likelihood of developing high blood pressure, which is a key risk factor for kidney disease.

Juicing can also help prevent kidney disease by providing the body with critical vitamins and minerals such as vitamin C, potassium, and magnesium. These nutrients are essential for keeping healthy kidneys and can help avoid the progression of renal disease. For example, potassium regulates fluid balance in the body and can help avoid fluid buildup, which is a common indication of kidney illness.

Finally, juicing can help avoid kidney disease by increasing hydration. Hydration is necessary for healthy kidney function, and consuming a diet rich in water-rich fruits and vegetables, such as through juicing, can help keep the body hydrated and support kidney health.

Juicing can help slow the progression of kidney disease and enhance overall health. It helps prevent kidney illness and enhance kidney function by providing the body with needed nutrients, decreasing toxic chemicals, and boosting hydration. However, before beginning a juicing plan,

Juicing for Kidney Health

consult with a healthcare physician because some fruits and vegetables can mix with certain drugs and have a detrimental effect on the kidneys.

Benefits of juicing for kidney health.

Juicing is a popular way to consume a significant amount of fruits and vegetables in a handy and delicious manner. Fruits and vegetables provide nutrients that can help kidney health in a variety of ways, including:

Hydration: Juicing can boost fluid consumption, which is necessary for maintaining good kidney function. This can aid in the prevention of dehydration, which is a major issue in people with kidney disease.

Fruits and vegetables are high in antioxidants, which can help reduce inflammation and oxidative stress in the kidneys. This can help protect the kidneys and reduce the progression of renal disease.

Vitamins and minerals: Fruits and vegetables are high in vitamins and minerals, such as vitamins C and E, potassium, magnesium, and iron. These nutrients are critical for overall health, including kidney health.

Anti-inflammatory Components: Many fruits and vegetables contain anti-inflammatory compounds, such as anthocyanin and flavonoids, which can help reduce inflammation in the kidneys.

Low Sodium: Juicing can help reduce sodium intake, which is crucial for managing high blood pressure and preventing kidney damage.

Low Protein: People with advanced renal disease should reduce their protein consumption to avoid further kidney damage. Juicing can provide a low-protein supply of vital nutrients without the extra protein.

Increased Fruit and Vegetable Intake: Juicing can help boost total fruit and vegetable intake, which is crucial for overall health and preventing chronic diseases like kidney disease.

Juicing for Kidney Health

It is crucial to realize that not all juices are made equal, and some can be heavy in sugar, preservatives, and artificial sweeteners, which can be harmful to kidney health. To assure the finest quality and health-promoting advantages, create fresh juices at home from a variety of colorful fruits and vegetables.

Juicing can have various benefits for kidney health, including improved hydration, antioxidants, vitamins, minerals, anti-inflammatory chemicals, low salt, and increased fruit and vegetable intake. However, it is critical to create fresh juices at home from a variety of colorful fruits and vegetables to ensure the greatest quality and health-promoting nutrients.

To summarize, knowing renal health issues and the role of juicing in maintaining kidney function is critical for overall health and wellness. Kidneys filter waste products and excess fluids from the blood, manage electrolyte balance, and produce hormones that control blood pressure and red blood cell development. Chronic Kidney Disease (CKD) is a silent and progressing disorder that can cause a slew of symptoms and problems if not treated properly.

Juicing can have various benefits for kidney health, including improved hydration, antioxidants, vitamins and minerals, anti-inflammatory chemicals, low salt, and increased fruit and vegetable intake. However, it is critical to create fresh juices at home from a variety of colorful fruits and vegetables to ensure the greatest quality and health-promoting nutrients. Regular check-ups with a healthcare professional, maintaining healthy lifestyle choices, and controlling underlying medical issues can help preserve kidney function and prevent the advancement of renal disease.

In conclusion, taking care of our kidneys is a crucial aspect of maintaining overall health and wellness, and understanding the relevance of renal health issues and the role of juicing in supporting kidney function can help us make informed health decisions.

Juicing for Kidney Health

CHAPTER 3

Karen, a 45-year-old lady, had been feeling weariness, swelling in her feet, and problems sleeping. She was diagnosed with early-stage Chronic Kidney Disease (CKD) after seeing her doctor, and she was advised she needed to make significant adjustments to her diet and lifestyle to prevent the progression of her ailment.

Karen was determined to take control of her health, so she began investigating various techniques to boost her kidney function. That's when she learned the benefits of juicing for renal health. She discovered that juicing might aid her hydration, provide her with critical vitamins and minerals, and boost her body's natural ability to remove waste and pollutants.

Karen began creating fresh juices at home with a range of colorful fruits and vegetables, such as beets, carrots, apples, and leafy greens. She also included fruits and vegetables high in antioxidants, anti-inflammatory chemicals, and low in salt, all of which are favorable to kidney function. In addition to juicing, Karen altered her diet by limiting her intake of processed foods and increasing her intake of nutritious grains, lean proteins, and healthy fats.

Karen found major improvements in her energy levels, sleep, and swelling after introducing juicing into her daily routine and making other dietary changes. She also underwent frequent doctor check-ups and was relieved to learn that her kidney function had stabilized and her CKD was no longer developing.

Juicing is a trendy practice that has grown in popularity in recent years as more individuals explore ways to improve their health and wellness. While juicing is frequently associated with weight loss, detoxification, and improved digestion, it can also be an excellent strategy to support kidney health. The kidneys filter waste products and excess fluids from the blood, manage electrolyte balance, and produce hormones that control blood pressure and red blood cell development. Maintaining excellent kidney function is critical for general health, but with chronic kidney disease (CKD) affecting millions of people worldwide, understanding the principles of juicing for kidney health has never been more important.

Juicing for Kidney Health

It is an easy and practical way to consume a range of fruits and vegetables that are high in vitamins, minerals, and antioxidants that can help support kidney function and prevent the advancement of renal disease. Juicing can help promote hydration and provide the body with important nutrients that are easily absorbed by the body by breaking down fruits and vegetables into liquid form.

In this chapter, we will look at the fundamentals of juicing for kidney health and how including fresh juices into our diet can assist, support, and improve kidney function. We will also explore the benefits of juicing for kidney health, the finest fruits and vegetables for kidney health, and how to include juicing into our daily routine. Whether you want to preserve decent kidney function, delay the progression of CKD, or simply enhance your general health and well-being, the foundations of juicing for kidney health are a crucial part of a healthy and balanced lifestyle.

IMPORTANCE OF HYDRATION FOR KIDNEY HEALTH

Hydration is essential for the kidneys to function properly. The kidneys are in charge of filtering waste and surplus fluids from the blood and excreting them from the body as urine. Adequate fluid consumption helps to ensure that the kidneys work effectively and minimizes the risk of kidney disorders such as kidney stones and chronic kidney disease.

Juicing is a convenient and tasty technique to boost fluid intake and support kidney function. It is an excellent way to hydrate the body because of the high water content of many fruits and vegetables used in juicing, such as cucumbers, celery, and watermelon. Furthermore, the fluid content of freshly prepared juice is quickly absorbed by the body, resulting in rapid hydration.

Incorporating juicing into a daily routine can also assist in improving total fluid consumption and encourage people to drink more water and other hydrating beverages. If you struggle to drink enough water, adding a tasty and nutrient-rich juice to your daily routine can help.

It is crucial to realize that not all juices are similarly hydrated. Some juices, such as those produced from high-sugar fruits, might have a diuretic effect and cause excessive fluid loss. As a result, it is critical to choose juicing ingredients that are both hydrating and beneficial to kidney health.

Juicing for Kidney Health

Hydration is critical for maintaining good kidney function and lowering the risk of kidney diseases. Juicing is a simple and pleasant technique to boost fluid consumption and promote kidney health, as long as the correct components are used. It is usually important to speak with a healthcare practitioner before beginning a juicing regimen, especially if you have any current kidney problems.

Nutrient-dense.

Juicing is a way of extracting the juice from fruits and vegetables to make a concentrated drink high in vitamins, minerals, and phytochemicals. These nutrients are vital for overall health and well-being, but they are especially important for kidney health.

Vitamins and minerals are necessary for the normal functioning of the body and play an important role in sustaining kidney health. Vitamin C, for example, protects the kidneys from oxidative stress damage, while Vitamin B6 helps to maintain proper renal function. Magnesium is also beneficial to kidney health since it helps regulate blood pressure and prevent the production of kidney stones.

Phytochemicals are plant-based substances that have been found to offer a variety of health benefits, including lowering the risk of chronic diseases such as kidney disease. Flavonoids, for example, have been found to protect the kidneys by lowering inflammation and oxidative stress. Carotenoids, another type of phytochemical, have also been found to improve kidney health by increasing blood flow to the kidneys and decreasing oxidative stress.

Juicing helps you consume a high amount of essential nutrients in a concentrated manner. This implies that you can get a lot of vitamins, minerals, and phytochemicals in a single dose, making it easier to achieve your daily nutritional needs. Furthermore, because the juice is swiftly absorbed into the bloodstream, the nutrients can be given directly to the kidneys, where they can be put to work supporting their health and function.

While juicing can be a terrific method to enhance your consumption of vitamins, minerals, and phytochemicals, it is not a replacement for a nutritious diet that includes a variety of whole fruits and vegetables. Furthermore, it is critical to use a balanced blend of fruits and vegetables in your

Juicing for Kidney Health

juice, as some fruits and vegetables are high in sugar and may not be suitable for people with renal disease.

To summarize, juicing is an easy and practical approach to eating a high quantity of vitamins, minerals, and phytochemicals in a concentrated form, which is crucial for maintaining kidney health. However, it is critical to consume a diverse range of fruits and vegetables rather than relying primarily on juicing to receive these essential elements.

Antioxidants for kidney protection.

Antioxidants are chemicals that serve to protect the body from the effects of oxidative stress. Oxidative stress occurs when there is an imbalance between the generation of reactive oxygen species (ROS) and the body's ability to neutralize these damaging molecules. ROS can harm cells, tissues, and organs, including the kidneys.

The kidneys are especially vulnerable to oxidative stress because they are constantly exposed to high amounts of blood flow, which can generate a considerable amount of ROS. Chronic kidney disease is a typical outcome of oxidative stress and inflammation in the kidneys.

Antioxidants can assist to protect the kidneys from oxidative stress damage by neutralizing ROS before they cause injury. Vitamins C and E, as well as carotenoids such as beta-carotene, are among the most significant antioxidants for kidney function. These antioxidants are abundant in many fruits and vegetables, making a diet rich in these foods a vital role in preserving kidney function.

Fruits and vegetables are also high in phytochemicals with antioxidant characteristics, such as flavonoids, phenols, and anthocyanins. These substances synergistically protect the kidneys from oxidative stress when eaten together.

Antioxidants are critical in protecting the kidneys from oxidative stress and injury. A diet high in antioxidants, such as fruits and vegetables, can assist to preserve kidney function and minimize the risk of chronic renal disease. You can help your kidneys operate correctly by include a range of antioxidant-rich foods in your diet.

Juicing for Kidney Health

Choosing low-potassium and low-phosphorus foods.

Avoiding high-potassium and high-phosphorus diets is vital for those with renal difficulties to maintain kidney health and prevent further kidney damage. The kidneys play an important role in managing the amounts of potassium and phosphorus in the body, and when the kidneys are not operating properly, these levels can become excessive, which can be harmful to health.

Hyperkalemia is a disorder caused by high amounts of potassium in the blood, which can lead to heart problems, muscle weakness, and other health issues. High phosphorus levels can also create health problems, such as the formation of kidney stones and an increased risk of cardiovascular disease.

When juicing, consider low-potassium and low-phosphorus choices to prevent raising these levels in the body. Lettuce, kale, spinach, cucumber, and celery are among the best low-potassium and low-phosphorus fruits and vegetables for juicing. These alternatives are also low in sugar and calories, making them excellent for people with renal disease who need to limit their sugar and calorie intake.

Avoiding high-potassium and high-phosphorus foods is critical for those with kidney difficulties in order to maintain kidney health and prevent additional damage. When juicing, consider low-potassium and low-phosphorus choices to prevent raising these levels in the body and to provide the kidneys with the support they require to function effectively.

Types of juicers.

There are various varieties of juicers available, each with their own set of advantages and disadvantages. The following are the most common types of juicers:

Centrifugal Juicers: Centrifugal juicers are the most prevalent type of juicer and are noted for their low cost and ease of operation. They work by shredding fruits and vegetables with a high-speed rotating blade and then separating the juice from the pulp using a sieve. Centrifugal juicers are often quick and efficient, making them an excellent choice for individuals who are short on time.

Pros: affordability, speed, efficiency, and ease of use.

Juicing for Kidney Health

Cons: It can heat up the juice, is not as effective with leafy greens, and produces less juice than masticating juicers.

Masticating Juicers: Masticating juicers, also known as slow juicers, extract juice from fruits and vegetables using a slower speed and a gentle chewing motion. This method is slower than a centrifugal juicer, but it yields more juice with more nutritional value since it reduces oxidation and heat accumulation.

Pros: high juice output, little oxidation, increased nutritional content, and the ability to handle leafy greens and other dense vegetables.

Cons: They are more expensive and slower than centrifugal juicers, and they are also more difficult to clean.

Triturating Juicers: Triturating juicers are similar to masticating juicers, but they extract juice using a dual-gear mechanism. This sort of juicer is designed to generate a high juice yield and is regarded as the most efficient type of juicer.

Pros: high juice output, little oxidation, increased nutritional content, and the ability to handle leafy greens and other dense vegetables.

Cons: It is the most expensive type of juicer, it is slower than centrifugal juicers, and it is the most difficult to clean.

Finally, while selecting a juicer, it is critical to consider your particular needs and preferences, such as the sorts of fruits and vegetables you want to juice, how frequently you will use the juicer, and your budget. Each type of juicer has advantages and disadvantages, so it is critical to research and evaluate your options before choosing which one is best for you.

Precautions and warnings.

When it comes to their eating and juicing habits, people with kidney difficulties should take some measures and be aware of some warnings.

Precautions:

Juicing for Kidney Health

Protein restriction: People with kidney difficulties should limit their protein consumption since their kidneys may have difficulty processing large amounts of protein.Consultation with a medical professional: Before beginning a juicing regimen, people with renal difficulties should check with a healthcare expert since several fruits and vegetables are high in potassium or phosphorus, which can be detrimental to those with kidney problems.

Warnings:

Potassium levels are high in several fruits and vegetables, such as bananas, oranges, and potatoes, and can be detrimental to people with kidney difficulties. Phosphorus levels are high in several fruits and vegetables, such as dairy products, nuts, and legumes, and can be detrimental to people with kidney difficulties. Patients with kidney difficulties should be aware of their protein, potassium, and phosphorus intake and should contact a healthcare expert before beginning a juicing plan.

Including juice in a diet can provide numerous health benefits, but people with kidney problems should be cautious. People with kidney difficulties should limit their protein intake since their kidneys may have difficulty processing large amounts of protein. It is also critical for people with kidney problems to watch their potassium and phosphorus intake, as some fruits and vegetables are high in these minerals and can be harmful to those with kidney problems.

Before beginning a juicing regimen, those with kidney difficulties should contact a healthcare expert. A healthcare professional can make individualized suggestions based on the individual's specific health needs, as well as help monitor the individual's health and change the juicing routine as needed.

Furthermore, those with renal difficulties should be aware of the potential hazards and adhere to certain general guidelines when adding juice to their diet. This involves eating low-potassium and low-phosphorus fruits and vegetables, avoiding high-potassium and high-phosphorus fruits and vegetables, and limiting protein intake.

A consultation with a healthcare practitioner is strongly advised for people with kidney problems who want to incorporate juicing into their diet.

Juicing for Kidney Health

Juicing for Kidney Health

CHAPTER 4

The Benefits of Juicing for Kidney Health

Mary, a 55-year-old woman who was diagnosed with renal disease several years ago. Her doctor encouraged her to make dietary modifications to help her kidney health. She was initially overwhelmed and unsure of what to do, but was determined to find a method to improve her health.

She decided to give juicing for kidney health a try after hearing about the benefits. She began including fresh fruit and vegetable juices in her regular diet and was astounded by the excellent influence it had on her health.

Mary observed that her energy levels had grown and was feeling more alert and focused after only a few weeks. She was also able to better control her blood pressure, which had been a worry for her due to her kidney difficulties.

Her renal function improved over time. Her doctor was impressed with her progress and told her that the minerals and antioxidants included in the fruits and vegetables she was juicing were helping to maintain her kidney health and lower oxidative stress.

Mary was also relieved to discover that by introducing plant-based protein sources into her juices, she was able to lessen her protein intake, which was putting a burden on her kidneys. This not only reduced the stress on her kidneys, but it also improved her general health.

Overall, she was grateful for the excellent influence juicing had on her kidney health. Every day, she was able to drink a variety of fresh and nutrient-rich juices, which helped to strengthen her kidney function and improve her general well-being. She would certainly recommend juicing to anyone with kidney difficulties searching for a natural and enjoyable alternative to support their health.

Juicing has become widely known in recent years, with many individuals incorporating fresh fruit and vegetable juices into their meals for enhanced health and wellness.

Juicing for Kidney Health

Fresh fruit and vegetable juices can provide a concentrated source of key vitamins, minerals, and antioxidants that are beneficial for kidney health. Juicing can also help minimize the workload on the kidneys by breaking down the fruits and vegetables into a form that is easier for the kidneys to digest.

Juicing can also help lower blood pressure, stimulate the immune system, maintain an alkaline balance in the body, reduce inflammation, raise energy levels, and improve mood. These advantages can be especially beneficial to those who have kidney difficulties in terms of supporting their health and increasing their quality of life.

When introducing juicing into their diet, those with renal difficulties must be aware of their protein, potassium, and phosphorus intake. It is also important to check with a healthcare practitioner before beginning a juicing plan to ensure that the individual's specific health needs are satisfied.

Here, we will look at the benefits of juicing for kidney health, such as increased hydration, increased nutrient intake, reduced stress on the kidneys, improved kidney function, blood pressure control, antioxidant support, a boosted immune system, alkaline balance, reduced inflammation, and increased energy and mood. Juicing can be a delicious and convenient approach to reaching your health objectives, whether you want to improve your kidney health or simply add more fruits and vegetables to your diet.

Improved Hydration.

Improved hydration is critical for people who have kidney problems because it helps to flush out toxins and waste products from the body, reducing stress on the kidneys. The kidneys rely on an appropriate flow of fluid to filter waste and sustain proper renal function. When the body is dehydrated, the kidneys have to work harder to filter waste, causing increased stress on the kidneys and potentially renal damage over time.

Juicing is a simple and practical technique to boost fluid consumption and enhance hydration. Most fruit and vegetable juices are rich in water content and can be a delightful and hydrating

Juicing for Kidney Health

supplement to the diet. Furthermore, many fruits and vegetables include critical vitamins and minerals that can help promote kidney health and prevent oxidative stress.

Cucumber, watermelon, celery, apples, and grapes are all good choices for people with renal difficulties.

Fruit juices should also be avoided because they are high in sugar and may aggravate kidney problems in some people. Vegetable juices are often a better choice because they contain less sugar and are higher in nutrients that support kidney health.

In conclusion, juicing can be an easy and comfortable way to boost fluid consumption and enhance hydration, which is critical for people with kidney difficulties. People with renal difficulties can improve their kidney health and minimize oxidative stress by introducing fresh fruit and vegetable juices into their diets while also enjoying a delightful and hydrating drink. To support optimal kidney health, contact a healthcare practitioner before beginning a juicing regimen and choose juices low in potassium, phosphorus, and protein.

Boosted Nutrient Intake.

Fruits and vegetables are an important source of vitamins, minerals, and antioxidants that promote general health, which is especially important for those with renal difficulties. The kidneys filter waste and excess fluids from the body, and a diet that promotes kidney health can improve overall health.

Juicing allows people with kidney difficulties to consume a range of fruits and vegetables in concentrated form, increasing their vitamin intake. Juicing breaks down fruits and vegetables into a form that is easier for the body to absorb, delivering a concentrated amount of critical nutrients.

Fresh fruit and vegetable juices can provide a concentrated source of key vitamins, minerals, and antioxidants that are beneficial for kidney health. For example, vitamin C, which is found in many fruits and vegetables, is a powerful antioxidant that can help to minimize oxidative stress and improve kidney function. Similarly, vitamin K, which is present in leafy greens, can help lower the risk of kidney disease by reducing oxidative stress and inflammation.

Juicing for Kidney Health

Fruits and vegetables are high in phytochemicals, which are natural compounds that have been demonstrated to protect the kidneys. These substances can help to minimize oxidative stress, improve kidney function, and lower the risk of renal disease.

Juicing allows people with kidney difficulties to consume a range of fruits and vegetables in concentrated form, increasing their vitamin intake. People with renal difficulties can enhance their general well-being by including fresh fruit and vegetable juices in their meals. To ensure maximum health, choose juices low in potassium, phosphorus, and protein, and speak with a healthcare expert before beginning a juicing plan.

Reduced Stress on the Kidneys.

The kidneys filter waste and excess fluids from the body, and a diet that promotes kidney health can improve overall health. People with kidney problems are frequently advised to limit their use of specific foods and beverages, as some might place a burden on the kidneys and exacerbate kidney disorders.

Juicing can help lessen the stress on the kidneys by breaking down fruits and vegetables into a form that is easier for the kidneys to digest. When we eat fruits and vegetables, the body must first break them down into a form that can be absorbed and used by the body. This process can be taxing on the kidneys, since they must struggle to filter the waste products created during digestion.

By consuming fruits and vegetables in concentrated form via juicing, the body can absorb the important nutrients more quickly, minimizing the stress on the kidneys. Juicing also helps to boost fluid consumption, which is crucial for those with kidney difficulties since it helps to flush out toxins and waste products from the body, lowering stress on the kidneys.Before beginning juicing, consult with a healthcare expert.

Finally, it can help minimize the stress on the kidneys by breaking down fruits and vegetables into a form that is easier for the kidneys to digest. People with renal difficulties can improve their kidney health and minimize stress on their kidneys by introducing fresh fruit and vegetable juices

Juicing for Kidney Health

into their diets while also enjoying a delightful and refreshing drink. To ensure maximum health, choose juices low in potassium, phosphorus, and protein, and speak with a healthcare expert before beginning a juicing plan.

Improved Kidney Function.

Renal function is vital for overall health and well-being, and a diet that promotes healthy kidney function can benefit the body. People with renal difficulties may have symptoms such as weariness, muscle weakness, and difficulty concentrating, which can have a substantial impact on their quality of life.

Juicing can assist in maintaining healthy kidney function by supplying critical vitamins, minerals, and antioxidants. Fruits and vegetables are high in these nutrients, and juicing them allows the body to absorb them more quickly.

Vitamins, such as Vitamin C, can help protect the kidneys from injury, while minerals, such as magnesium and potassium, are crucial for maintaining good blood pressure levels and fluid balance in the body, all of which can benefit renal function. Antioxidants, such as Vitamin E and beta-carotene, can help protect the kidneys from oxidative stress and prevent kidney disease.

Control of Blood Pressure.

Renal function is vital for overall health and well-being, and a diet that promotes healthy kidney function can benefit the body. People with renal difficulties may have symptoms such as weariness, muscle weakness, and difficulty concentrating, which can have a substantial impact on their quality of life.

Juicing can assist in maintaining healthy kidney function by supplying critical vitamins, minerals, and antioxidants. People with renal difficulties can enhance their general well-being by including fresh fruit and vegetable juices in their meals.

Juicing for Kidney Health

On a daily basis, the kidneys are subjected to severe oxidative stress and damage, which can lead to a reduction in renal function over time. Antioxidants are critical for protecting the kidneys from oxidative stress and damage, and a high-antioxidant diet can help support healthy kidney function.

Juicing can provide a concentrated amount of antioxidants, allowing patients with renal difficulties to enjoy a range of fruits and vegetables. Antioxidants like Vitamin E and beta-carotene can help protect the kidneys from oxidative stress and prevent kidney disease.

Furthermore, many fruits and vegetables include antioxidants such as polyphenols and anthocyanins that are difficult to obtain from other dietary sources. Berries, for example, are high in antioxidants such as anthocyanins, which have been demonstrated to protect the kidneys.

It is critical to be aware of the ingredients used in juices, as some fruits and vegetables have high levels of potassium, phosphorus, and protein, which can strain the kidneys. It is advisable to choose juices that are low in these nutrients and to consult with a healthcare practitioner before beginning a juicing plan to ensure that you are not deficient in these nutrients.

Boosted Immune System

The human immune system is a complex network of cells, tissues, and organs that work together to protect the body from diseases and outside invaders. A compromised immune system can make an individual more susceptible to infections and illnesses, which can be especially problematic for those with kidney difficulties, as their health condition may already be affecting their ability to fight infections.

It helps improve the immune system by supplying the body with a concentrated dosage of important vitamins, minerals, and antioxidants. Citrus fruits, berries, leafy greens, and carrots, for example, are high in vitamin C, which has been shown to promote immunological function. Furthermore, many of these same foods are high in additional nutrients such as beta-carotene, folate, and iron, which all play significant roles in immune system health.

Juicing for Kidney Health

It is crucial to stress, however, that juicing should not be viewed as a miracle cure for boosting the immune system. A well-balanced diet rich in fruits, vegetables, whole grains, and lean meats is still the best way to support general health, including immunological function. Additionally, before making any big changes to your diet, consult with your doctor, especially if you have a pre-existing health condition such as kidney problems.

Alkaline Balance.

The pH level of the body is referred to as the "alkaline balance," with 7.0 being the neutral pH. An alkaline environment is one with a pH above 7.0, whereas an acidic environment has a pH below 7.0. The human body is naturally constructed to maintain a slightly alkaline pH, and this balance is critical for overall health and well-being.

An acidic environment can place additional strain on the kidneys, which are crucial in regulating the body's pH level. The kidneys serve to filter waste items from the bloodstream and eliminate excess acids from the body through urine. When the body becomes overly acidic, the kidneys must work harder to maintain a good pH balance, which can put additional strain on the already impaired kidneys of those with kidney disorders.

It helps maintain an alkaline balance in the body by supplying the body with a concentrated dosage of alkaline-forming foods such as leafy greens, vegetables, and certain fruits. These foods provide critical vitamins, minerals, and antioxidants that can help neutralize excess acids in the body and support the kidneys in their efforts to maintain a healthy pH balance.

For example, leafy greens like spinach, kale, and lettuce are abundant in chlorophyll, which has a powerful alkalizing effect on the body. Similarly, foods like cucumbers, tomatoes, and celery are alkaline-forming and can help to offset the acidifying effects of a typical Western diet high in processed foods and animal products.

It's crucial to remember that juicing is only one component of a healthy diet and lifestyle, and it should not be used as a solitary source of nutrients. A well-balanced diet rich in fruits, vegetables, whole grains, and lean proteins is still the best way to promote general health,

Juicing for Kidney Health

including alkaline balance. Additionally, before making any big changes to your diet, consult with your doctor, especially if you have a pre-existing health condition such as kidney problems.

Reduced Inflammation.

Inflammation is a natural mechanism in the body that helps to guard against diseases and injuries. Chronic inflammation, in which the body's immune system becomes overactive and inflammation persists for long periods of time, can be damaging and contribute to a variety of health concerns, including kidney damage.

People with renal disorders are more vulnerable to the detrimental effects of inflammation since their kidneys are already damaged and working harder to accomplish their regular duties. This additional stress can leave the kidneys more susceptible to further injury and increase the risk of chronic kidney disease.

It reduces inflammation in the body by supplying the body with a concentrated dose of anti-inflammatory chemicals such as antioxidants, vitamins, and minerals. Berries, leafy greens, and turmeric, for example, include significant levels of antioxidants such as anthocyanins, flavonoids, and curcumin, which have been demonstrated to decrease inflammation and protect against cellular damage.

Furthermore, many of these same foods are high in critical vitamins and minerals, such as vitamin C and magnesium, which have anti-inflammatory qualities and play important roles in supporting a healthy immune system. By including these nutrients in your diet through juicing, you can help reduce inflammation and promote the health of your kidneys.

Remember that juicing isn't a miracle cure for inflammation. A well-balanced diet rich in fruits, vegetables, whole grains, and lean proteins is still the best strategy to improve overall health and reduce chronic inflammation. Additionally, before making any big changes to your diet, consult with your doctor, especially if you have a pre-existing health condition such as kidney problems.

Juicing for Kidney Health

Increased Energy and Improved Mood.

The quality and nutrients of the meals we eat can have a significant impact on our energy levels and mood. Because of their health condition, people with kidney difficulties may experience exhaustion and a decreased sense of well-being, making it harder to maintain a healthy and active lifestyle.

It boosts energy levels and improve mood by providing the body with a concentrated amount of vitamins, minerals, and antioxidants that are essential for overall health and well-being. Fruits and vegetables such as beets, leafy greens, and citrus fruits, for example, are high in natural sources of energy such as glucose as well as vitamins B and C, which are vital for energy metabolism and a healthy nervous system.

Aside from providing an energy boost, certain juice ingredients can also help with mood management and general well-being. For example, spinach and kale are high in folic acid, which has been demonstrated to help regulate mood and lessen depression symptoms. Similarly, meals high in antioxidants, such as berries and dark leafy greens, can help to protect against cellular damage and lower inflammation, which has been related to a decreased sense of well-being.

It should be viewed as one component of a balanced diet and lifestyle, not as a sole source of nutrients. A well-balanced diet rich in fruits, vegetables, whole grains, and lean meats remains the best method to promote general health, including energy levels and mood. Furthermore, before making any big changes to your diet, consult with your doctor, especially if you have a pre-existing health condition such as kidney problems.

In conclusion, juicing can be a beneficial and healthy supplement to the diet of those suffering from kidney disease. Juicing can promote kidney health and function in a variety of ways by giving the body a concentrated dosage of vital vitamins, minerals, and antioxidants.

Juicing, for example, can help enhance the immune system, maintain an alkaline balance in the body, reduce inflammation, increase energy levels, and improve mood. These benefits are especially important for people with kidney difficulties since their immune systems may be compromised, their bodies may be more vulnerable to inflammation, and they may experience exhaustion and a decreased sense of well-being as a result of their health condition.

Juicing for Kidney Health

However, it is crucial to remember that juicing is only one component of a balanced diet and lifestyle. A well-balanced diet rich in fruits, vegetables, whole grains, and lean proteins is still the best way to support general health and kidney health. Additionally, before making any big changes to your diet, consult with your doctor, especially if you have a pre-existing health condition such as kidney problems.

Juicing for Kidney Health

CHAPTER 5

Essential Nutrients for Kidney Health.

Kelvin is a 45-year-old guy who has had kidney difficulties for several years. Kelvin felt exhausted and worn down most of the time, despite following a tight treatment plan and taking his medications as directed. His doctor advised him to concentrate on including more important nutrients in his diet in order to improve his kidney function and overall well-being.

Kelvin chose to start juicing to obtain a concentrated dose of critical vitamins, minerals, and antioxidants in his diet. He began by juicing a range of fruits and vegetables, such as leafy greens, beets, berries, and citrus fruits. He was astounded at how soon he noticed an improvement in his energy levels and overall sense of well-being.

One of the most noticeable advantages Kelvin saw was an improvement in his immune system. He was able to bolster his immune system and lower his risk of infections and diseases by getting a concentrated dosage of vitamins and antioxidants from his juices. He was particularly pleased with the reduction in inflammation, which had been a key cause of his kidney troubles.

Kelvin also noticed an improvement in his mood and more energy throughout the day. His juices' important vitamins and minerals, such as vitamin B and folic acid, were critical in regulating his mood and giving him the energy he needed to stay active and engaged.

While juicing did not cure Kelvin's renal problems, it did play an important role in making him feel better and improving his overall health. He was delighted to have discovered a simple and handy approach to providing his body with the vital nutrients it required to support his kidney health and overall well-being.

The kidneys are an essential element of our systems, filtering waste and excess fluids, regulating blood pressure, and creating hormones that regulate red blood cells and keep bones strong. However, many people with renal disorders struggle to maintain excellent kidney health, typically due to a lack of necessary nutrients in their diets.

Providing the body with the vitamins, minerals, and antioxidants it needs can be a simple and effective strategy to support kidney health and general well-being. Vitamins B and C, potassium,

Juicing for Kidney Health

magnesium, and antioxidants such as flavonoids and carotenoids are among the most critical nutrients for kidney function.

While it is feasible to obtain these necessary elements via a balanced diet that includes a range of fruits, vegetables, whole grains, and lean proteins, some people may find it difficult to consume enough of these nutrients on a regular basis. This is where juicing can come in handy as a quick and healthy way to get a concentrated dose of essential nutrients into the body.

In this chapter, we will look at the benefits of including vital nutrients in your diet to promote kidney health, as well as some of the most nutritious items to include in your juices to maximize the benefits. Whether you have kidney difficulties or simply want to improve your general health and well-being, including important nutrients in your diet can be a simple and effective method to reach your goals.

Different types of essential nutrients.

The human body requires a variety of vital nutrients to function properly, and these nutrients are critical in sustaining kidney health. Vitamins, minerals, and antioxidants are all essential nutrients that are required in varying levels to support various physiological functions in the body.

Vitamins are chemical molecules that the body needs in little amounts to maintain diverse processes. Vitamins B and C are vital for kidney health because they help to produce red blood cells, regulate blood pressure, and support the immune system.

Minerals, on the other hand, are inorganic molecules that are needed in greater quantities than vitamins. Potassium and magnesium are two of the most important minerals for kidney health because they help regulate blood pressure and keep bones strong.

Antioxidants, such as flavonoids and carotenoids, play an important role in protecting the kidneys against oxidative stress and inflammation. Antioxidants neutralize free radicals, which are unstable chemicals that can cause cellular damage and lead to chronic kidney disease and other kidney disorders.

Juicing for Kidney Health

Incorporating these vital nutrients into your diet through a balanced and diverse diet, as well as juicing, can be an effective method to maintain kidney health and lower the risk of chronic kidney disease and other renal disorders. Leafy greens, beets, berries, and citrus fruits, which are high in vitamins, minerals, and antioxidants, are some of the most nutritious items to include in your juices for kidney health.

Overall, the many types of vital nutrients play an important role in sustaining renal health and preventing kidney diseases. By integrating these critical nutrients into your diet, you can help maintain normal kidney function and lower your risk of chronic renal disease and other kidney disorders.

Lack of essential nutrients can impact kidney health.

A lack of necessary nutrients can have major consequences for kidney health and raise the risk of kidney disorders, including chronic kidney disease. When the body is low in certain vitamins, minerals, and antioxidants, it can negatively affect various physiological systems, leading to a variety of health concerns.

Increased oxidative stress and inflammation are two of the most serious effects of a lack of key nutrients on kidney health. When the body lacks antioxidants, it becomes more vulnerable to free radical damage, which can cause cellular damage and contribute to the development of chronic kidney disease. Inflammation can also be increased by a lack of vital nutrients, increasing the risk of kidney injury.

Aside from increased oxidative stress and inflammation, a lack of vital nutrients can have an influence on blood pressure regulation, which is critical for keeping healthy kidneys. When the body lacks important minerals like potassium and magnesium, it can cause high blood pressure, which is a major risk factor for chronic kidney disease.

A lack of vital vitamins can potentially have major consequences for renal health. A shortage of vitamin B, for example, can cause anemia, which puts additional strain on the kidneys and increases the risk of renal disorders.

Juicing for Kidney Health

It is critical to remember that some people with chronic renal disease may also suffer from malnutrition, which can result from the kidneys' inability to digest nutrients effectively. This can enhance the risk of a shortage of key nutrients and increase the chance of kidney disorders.

In conclusion, a lack of vital nutrients can have major consequences for renal health and raise the likelihood of kidney issues, including chronic kidney disease. Incorporating a balanced and varied diet, as well as vital nutrients through juicing or supplements, is critical for maintaining excellent kidney health and lowering the risk of renal diseases.

The most nutritious ingredients to include in your juices for kidney health.

Incorporating nutritious components into your juices is an effective method to maintain kidney health and lower your risk of chronic kidney disease and other kidney disorders. Leafy greens, beets, berries, and citrus fruits are among the most nutritious ingredients to incorporate in your juices for kidney health.

Leafy greens, such as kale, spinach, and Swiss chard, are high in vitamins, minerals, and antioxidants, which are crucial for kidney health. Leafy greens are particularly rich in vitamins B and C, as well as magnesium, potassium, and antioxidants such as flavonoids. These nutrients are essential for regulating blood pressure, generating red blood cells, strengthening the immune system, and neutralizing free radicals, making leafy greens a good element for kidney health.

Beets are another nutritional item that is great for kidney health. Beets are high in antioxidants and anti-inflammatory chemicals, making them an ideal ingredient for lowering oxidative stress and inflammation. Beets are also high in folate, potassium, and magnesium, which are necessary for blood pressure regulation and bone health.

Berries, including blueberries, raspberries, and blackberries, are also great for kidney health. Berries are rich in antioxidants, such as flavonoids and carotenoids, which play an important role in neutralizing free radicals and lowering oxidative stress. Berries are particularly abundant in vitamins C and K, as well as magnesium and potassium, making them a good nutrient for kidney health.

Juicing for Kidney Health

Citrus fruits, such as lemons, limes, and oranges, are also high in vital elements that promote kidney function. Citrus fruits are abundant in vitamin C, which is vital for immune system support and free radical neutralization. Citrus fruits are also high in potassium, which is vital for blood pressure regulation and bone health.

Overall, these ingredients are high in critical vitamins, minerals, and antioxidants, which are crucial for supporting kidney health and lowering the risk of chronic kidney disease and other renal disorders. By including these nutritious nutrients in your juices, you can help support normal kidney function and lower your risk of renal issues.

The role of vitamins B and C in supporting kidney health.

Vitamins B and C are essential for maintaining kidney health. To function properly, the human body requires a healthy mix of vitamins and minerals, and deficits in these nutrients can contribute to a variety of health concerns, including kidney-related difficulties.

The vitamin B complex, which includes B1, B2, B3, B5, B6, B7, B9, and B12, is required for red blood cell synthesis and blood pressure management. B vitamins are essential for the metabolism of carbs, lipids, and proteins, which aids in the production of energy for numerous biological processes.

B1 (thiamine) and B2 (riboflavin) are required for appropriate kidney function and red blood cell formation. B3 (niacin) aids in blood pressure regulation and nervous system health. B6 (pyridoxine) aids in the synthesis of red blood cells, hormone regulation, and immune system maintenance. B9 (folic acid) aids in the production of red blood cells and is required for normal cell division. B12 (cobalamin) promotes nervous system health and the production of red blood cells.

Vitamin C, commonly known as ascorbic acid, is a water-soluble vitamin that functions as an antioxidant, preventing cell damage. It is required for the manufacture of collagen, which is required for the health of blood vessels, particularly those in the kidneys. Vitamin C also aids in blood pressure regulation by increasing blood vessel flexibility and decreasing oxidative stress.

Juicing for Kidney Health

The kidneys are essential organs that filter waste from the blood and regulate electrolyte levels such as sodium and potassium. Chronic kidney disease (CKD) is caused by a steady decline in kidney function over time. Vitamin B and C deficiency have been associated with the development of CKD and other kidney-related issues, such as nephropathy, a kidney condition.

Finally, vitamins B and C play an important role in kidney health by regulating blood pressure, generating red blood cells, and sustaining general body health. It is critical to maintain a balanced diet and adequate intake of these vitamins to support kidney health and avoid the development of kidney-related diseases. Consult a healthcare physician for tailored vitamin and mineral recommendations to promote kidney health.

Benefits of minerals like potassium and magnesium.

Minerals have an important role in general health, including kidney health. Potassium and magnesium, in particular, are critical for preventing renal disorders and sustaining kidney function.

Potassium is a mineral that is necessary for optimal fluid balance in the body, blood pressure regulation, and heart and muscle function. Potassium is also important in preventing the formation of kidney stones, which is a common kidney disease. High potassium levels in the blood can damage the kidneys and cause major health problems, so maintaining a good balance is critical. A diet high in fruits, vegetables, and low-fat dairy products can help the body get the potassium it requires.

Magnesium is yet another mineral that is necessary for overall health, including kidney health. It aids in the maintenance of proper muscle and nerve function, the support of a healthy immune system, and the regulation of blood sugar levels. Magnesium is also necessary for bone health, preventing kidney stone development, and lowering the chance of developing renal disease. A diet rich in whole grains, nuts, and green leafy vegetables can help the body acquire the magnesium it requires.

Chronic kidney disease (CKD) is a common kidney issue caused by the steady deterioration of kidney function over time. This can result in a variety of health issues, such as anemia, high

Juicing for Kidney Health

blood pressure, and heart disease. Proper potassium and magnesium consumption has been demonstrated to lower the chance of developing CKD as well as aid in controlling symptoms in people who already have the condition.

Finally, minerals such as potassium and magnesium play an important role in promoting renal function and preventing kidney diseases. It is critical to eat a well-balanced diet that contains all of the nutrients your body requires, including these crucial minerals. However, before making any dietary changes, it is always best to speak with a healthcare provider, especially if you have a medical condition or take prescription drugs, as certain medications might interact with minerals and reduce their efficacy.

The role of antioxidants in reducing inflammation and oxidative stress in the kidneys.

Antioxidants are substances that protect cells from free radical damage. Free radicals are unstable molecules that can cause oxidative stress and contribute to a variety of health problems, including kidney disease. Flavonoids and carotenoids are two forms of antioxidants that help to reduce inflammation and oxidative stress in the kidneys.

Flavonoids are a type of antioxidant present in a variety of fruits, vegetables, and other plant-based meals. These substances contain anti-inflammatory and antioxidant effects, which aid in the protection of the kidneys. Flavonoids also have a favorable effect on blood flow, which can help the kidneys work better. Quercetin, catechins, and anthocyanins are some of the most well-known flavonoids.

Carotenoids are another type of antioxidant found in fruits and vegetables such as carrots, spinach, and red bell peppers. These chemicals are essential for lowering oxidative stress and inflammation in the body. Carotenoids have also been proven to enhance blood flow, which can have a good impact on kidney function. Beta-carotene, lutein, and zeaxanthin are some of the best-known carotenoids.

Chronic kidney disease (CKD) is a common kidney issue caused by the steady deterioration of kidney function over time. This can result in a variety of health issues, such as anemia, high

Juicing for Kidney Health

blood pressure, and heart disease. Antioxidants such as flavonoids and carotenoids have been found to reduce oxidative stress and inflammation in the kidneys, potentially slowing the progression of CKD and lowering the risk of other kidney-related diseases.

Finally, antioxidants such as flavonoids and carotenoids are important in decreasing inflammation and oxidative stress in the kidneys. A diet high in fruits, vegetables, and other plant-based foods can supply the antioxidants the body requires to promote kidney health and lower the risk of kidney-related diseases. However, before making any dietary changes, always discuss them with a healthcare provider, especially if you have a medical condition or take prescription drugs, as certain medications might interact with antioxidants and reduce their efficacy.

Balancing your diet.

A well-balanced diet is vital for general health, including kidney function. Consuming a variety of fruits, vegetables, whole grains, and lean meats provides the body with the nutrients it requires to function correctly and reduces the chance of health problems. However, for some people, getting all of the nutrients they require from their diet alone may be difficult, and integrating critical nutrients through juicing or supplements may be important.

Fruits and vegetables provide the body with a variety of necessary nutrients, such as vitamins, minerals, and antioxidants. These nutrients promote general health and help prevent disease, particularly kidney disease. Eating a variety of colored fruits and vegetables can offer the body a variety of critical nutrients, as each color indicates a different nutrient category.

Whole grains, such as whole wheat, brown rice, and quinoa, are also essential components of a healthy diet. Whole grains deliver fiber to the body, which can help regulate digestion and lower the risk of health concerns such as heart disease and diabetes. Whole grains also supply critical minerals to the body, such as B vitamins, iron, and magnesium.

Lean proteins, such as chicken, fish, and tofu, are also essential components of a healthy diet. These proteins supply the amino acids required by the body to create and repair tissues, as well

Juicing for Kidney Health

as to produce hormones and enzymes. Lean proteins also aid in the regulation of blood sugar levels and the prevention of health concerns such as heart disease and stroke.

In some situations, getting all of the nutrients you need from your food alone may be difficult, and integrating important nutrients through juicing or supplements may be necessary. Juicing can supply the body with a concentrated dosage of critical vitamins and minerals, while supplements can aid in replacing nutritional shortages.

In conclusion, proper kidney health is essential for general health and well-being. Adequate intake of important nutrients such as protein, calcium, phosphorus, and vitamins is critical for maintaining good kidney function. Protein is necessary for tissue growth and repair, but calcium and phosphorus are required for strong bones. Vitamins, notably vitamin D, aid in the regulation of calcium and phosphorus balance in the body.

It is crucial to note that, while these nutrients are important for kidney health, some of them can be consumed in excess, which can be damaging to the kidneys. To assess the proper intake of these essential nutrients based on individual needs and health status, it is advisable to speak with a healthcare provider or a qualified dietitian. A balanced diet, as well as staying hydrated and avoiding harmful habits such as excessive alcohol intake and smoking, can all contribute to excellent kidney health. Overall, we can maintain our overall health and well-being for years to come by taking care of our kidneys and consuming the critical minerals they require to work effectively.

Juicing for Kidney Health

CHAPTER 6

Common Ingredients for Juicing for Kidney Health

Hassan was a middle-aged man who had always been sedentary and enjoyed junk food. He smoked, had high blood pressure, and was overweight. He was often fatigued and had a headache, but he didn't think much of it until he was diagnosed with chronic renal disease one day. The news was a wake-up call for Hassan, who recognized he needed to make major lifestyle changes if he wanted to save his kidneys and his life.

His doctor advised him to begin juicing as a method to incorporate more fruits and vegetables into his diet and improve his kidney function. Hassan was at first hesitant, but he was desperate to improve his health, so he decided to give it a shot. He began by combining typical kidney-health-promoting components such as beets, carrots, ginger, lemon, and apples.

The taste of the juices did not appeal to him at first, but as he became accustomed to them, he began to enjoy them. He also experienced a boost in energy, fewer headaches, and cleaner skin. Hassan was astounded by how much better he felt and how quickly the benefits came. He was also relieved to find that his creatinine levels, which indicate renal function, had improved.

As Hassan continued to juice, he made additional lifestyle modifications. He quit smoking, lowered his salt intake, and began exercising on a daily basis. He also lost weight, which reduced the strain on his kidneys. Hassan was resolved to do whatever it took to safeguard and improve his kidneys.

Hassan has had chronic kidney disease for many years and continues to juice on a regular basis. He has also become a strong champion for healthy living, inspiring many of his friends and family members to follow suit. Hassan exemplifies how, with the correct mindset and a commitment to healthy living, anyone can improve their kidney health.

To summarize, juicing is a tasty and simple way to consume a range of fruits and vegetables that are good for kidney health. Common components such as beets, carrots, ginger, lemons, and apples can help promote kidney health and function. Hassan's story demonstrates that it is

Juicing for Kidney Health

possible to improve kidney function and live a happier life with the appropriate mindset and commitment to healthy living.

Juicing is a popular and convenient way to consume a range of nutritious fruits and vegetables. Certain components can help maintain the health and function of these vital organs when it comes to kidney health. Our kidneys filter waste and extra fluids from our bloodstream, so it's crucial to provide them with the nutrients they require to function effectively.

In this chapter, we will look at some of the most popular substances used in juicing for kidney health, as well as the benefits they provide. We'll look at how foods like beetroot and carrots, as well as ginger and lemon, can help maintain the health of our kidneys. Whether you want to add more fruits and vegetables to your diet or improve your general health, these common items are a wonderful place to start.

Common ingredients used in juicing for kidney health.

The following are ten common fruits that are frequently used in juicing to support kidney health:

Apples: Apples are high in antioxidants, fiber, and vitamin C, all of which improve kidney function and help to avoid kidney injury. Furthermore, apples are low in potassium and phosphorus, which can help alleviate kidney stress.

Blueberries: Blueberries are high in antioxidants and vitamins, which enhance kidney function. They are also low in potassium and phosphorus, making them an excellent alternative for those suffering from kidney disease.

Cranberries are well-known for their ability to prevent urinary tract infections, which can strain the kidneys. They are also high in antioxidants and vitamin C, both of which can help protect the kidneys from harm.

Grapefruits: High in antioxidants and vitamin C, grapefruits can help protect the kidneys from injury. They are also low in potassium and phosphorus, making them an excellent alternative for those suffering from kidney disease.

Juicing for Kidney Health

Lemons: Lemons are high in vitamin C, which is vital for immune system health, and they also help to alkalize the body, which is helpful for kidney health. Lemons are also poor in potassium and phosphorus.

Oranges are high in vitamin C and antioxidants, which can help protect the kidneys from harm. They are also low in potassium and phosphorus, making them an excellent alternative for those suffering from kidney disease.

Pears: Pears are high in fiber and low in potassium and phosphorus, which can help alleviate renal stress. Pears also include antioxidants and vitamin C, which can benefit kidney health.

Pineapple: Pineapple is high in antioxidants and vitamin C, which can benefit kidney function. It is also high in bromelain, an enzyme that aids in the breakdown of proteins and the prevention of kidney stones.

Strawberries are high in antioxidants, vitamin C, and fiber, all of which aid in maintaining kidney health. They are also low in potassium and phosphorus, making them an excellent choice for people who have kidney difficulties.

Watermelon: High in antioxidants and vitamin C, watermelon can help promote kidney health. It is also low in potassium and phosphorus, making it an excellent choice for people who have kidney difficulties.

Also, the following are common vegetables that are frequently used in juicing to support kidney health:

Beets: High in antioxidants and anti-inflammatory substances, beets can help protect the kidneys from injury. They are also low in potassium, making them an excellent alternative for patients suffering from kidney disease.

Carrots: High in antioxidants and vitamin A, carrots can help protect the kidneys from injury. They are also low in potassium, making them an excellent alternative for patients suffering from kidney disease.

Cucumbers: High in antioxidants and anti-inflammatory chemicals, cucumbers can help maintain kidney health. They are also low in potassium, making them an excellent choice for people who have kidney difficulties.

Juicing for Kidney Health

Leafy greens, such as spinach, kale, and collard greens, are high in antioxidants and vitamins that support kidney health. They are also low in potassium, making them an excellent choice for people who have kidney difficulties.

Celery is abundant in antioxidants and anti-inflammatory chemicals, which can benefit kidney function. It is also low in potassium, making it a suitable choice for people who have kidney difficulties.

Ginger: Ginger is well-known for its anti-inflammatory effects, which can help relieve renal stress. It is also abundant in antioxidants, which can help protect the kidneys from harm.

Garlic contains antioxidants and anti-inflammatory chemicals that can benefit kidney function. It has also been demonstrated to lessen the chance of getting kidney disease.

Parsley contains antioxidants and anti-inflammatory chemicals that can benefit kidney function. It is also low in potassium, making it a suitable choice for people who have kidney difficulties.

Peppers: Peppers, particularly red and yellow peppers, are abundant in antioxidants and vitamin C, which can help preserve the kidneys. They are also low in potassium, making them an excellent alternative for patients suffering from kidney disease.

Squash: Squash contains a lot of antioxidants and anti-inflammatory substances that can help with kidney function. It is also low in potassium, making it a suitable choice for people who have kidney difficulties.

Juicing is an excellent technique to improve kidney health and consume a range of nutrient-dense veggies. Include these ten common veggies in your juicing program to help support kidney function and prevent kidney injury. However, before making any big changes to your diet, you should consult with a healthcare physician, especially if you have a history of renal difficulties.

Incorporating these popular elements into your juicing program can help maintain your kidney's health and function. You can provide your body with the nutrients it requires to maintain good kidney function by consuming juices produced with these ingredients. While juicing might be a simple method to incorporate more fruits and vegetables into your diet, it is still vital to eat a balanced diet that includes a range of whole fruits and vegetables, lean protein, and whole grains.

Juicing for Kidney Health

Fruits and vegetables are an important element of a healthy diet since they provide the body with numerous benefits such as hydration, antioxidants and anti-inflammatory effects, vitamins and minerals, and soluble fiber.

Hydration: Many fruits and vegetables contain a lot of water, which helps the body stay hydrated. This is especially crucial for folks who may not drink enough water each day.

They are high in antioxidants and anti-inflammatory chemicals, which help protect the body from free radical damage and reduce inflammation.

Vitamins and minerals: Fruits and vegetables are high in vitamins and minerals, including vitamin C, vitamin A, potassium, and magnesium. These minerals are essential for overall health and illness prevention.

Soluble Fiber: Fruits and vegetables are high in soluble fiber, which aids in blood sugar regulation, heart health, and digestive health.

Let's take a closer look at each fruit and vegetable's advantages:

Beets: high in antioxidants and anti-inflammatory chemicals, as well as vitamins and minerals such as folate, manganese, and potassium. They are also abundant in soluble fiber, which can aid in blood sugar regulation.

Carrots include antioxidants and anti-inflammatory chemicals, as well as vitamins and minerals such as vitamin A, potassium, and magnesium. They're also high in soluble fiber, which can help manage blood sugar levels.

Cucumbers have significant levels of antioxidants and anti-inflammatory chemicals, as well as vitamins and minerals such as vitamin C, potassium, and magnesium. They are also an excellent source of hydration due to their high water content.

Leafy greens, such as spinach, kale, and collard greens, are high in antioxidants and anti-inflammatory chemicals, as well as vitamins and minerals such as vitamin C, vitamin A, and magnesium. They are also abundant in soluble fiber, which can aid in blood sugar regulation.

Juicing for Kidney Health

Celery contains antioxidants and anti-inflammatory chemicals, as well as vitamins and minerals such as vitamin C, potassium, and magnesium. It's also high in soluble fiber, which can help manage blood sugar levels.

Ginger is well-known for its anti-inflammatory effects, which can aid in the reduction of inflammation in the body. It also contains antioxidants, vitamins, and minerals such as potassium and magnesium.

Garlic contains antioxidants and anti-inflammatory chemicals, as well as vitamins and minerals such as vitamin C, manganese, and potassium. It's also high in soluble fiber, which can help manage blood sugar levels.

Parsley contains antioxidants and anti-inflammatory chemicals, as well as vitamins and minerals such as vitamin C, folate, and potassium. It's also high in soluble fiber, which can help manage blood sugar levels.

Peppers: Red and yellow peppers, in particular, are high in antioxidants and anti-inflammatory chemicals, as well as vitamins and minerals such as vitamin C, potassium, and magnesium. They're also high in soluble fiber, which can help manage blood sugar levels.

Squash contains a high concentration of antioxidants and anti-inflammatory chemicals, as well as vitamins and minerals such as vitamin C, potassium, and magnesium. It is also high in soluble fiber, which can aid in digestion.

Juicing ingredients help support the health and function of the kidneys.
The kidneys are essential for overall health because they filter waste materials from the blood and manage fluid balance in the body. A bad diet, stress, and disease, on the other hand, can cause renal malfunction and damage over time.

A diet high in fruits and vegetables can help to promote kidney health and function by supplying numerous nutrients and chemicals that are helpful to the kidneys. These components can aid in the following ways:

Juicing for Kidney Health

Toxin Removal: The kidneys filter waste products and toxins from the blood, and a diet rich in fruits and vegetables can help to support this process by giving necessary nutrients and chemicals to the kidneys. Some fruits and vegetables, such as beets, contain significant levels of antioxidants and anti-inflammatory chemicals, which can aid in the removal of toxins from the body and the reduction of oxidative stress.

Reducing Oxidative Stress: Oxidative stress is a state in which the body's free radicals and antioxidants are out of equilibrium. Cellular damage and an increased risk of disease, particularly kidney disease, can result from this. A diet high in antioxidants and anti-inflammatory substances, such as those found in leafy greens, carrots, and beets, can help minimize oxidative stress and protect the kidneys.

Improving Kidney Function: Cucumbers, celery, and ginger contain chemicals that have been found to increase renal function and lower the risk of kidney disease. Furthermore, many fruits and vegetables, such as garlic and parsley, are high in vitamins and minerals needed for kidney function, such as potassium and magnesium.

Blood Sugar Control: High blood sugar levels can be harmful to the kidneys, increasing the risk of kidney disease over time. Some fruits and vegetables, such as beets, carrots, and leafy greens, are high in soluble fiber, which aids in blood sugar regulation and prevents blood sugar spikes.

Maintaining Hydration: Hydration is essential for kidney health since it aids in the removal of waste products and the healthy functioning of the kidneys. A diet high in water-rich fruits and vegetables, such as cucumbers and watermelon, can assist in maintaining hydration and improving kidney function.

A diet high in fruits and vegetables can help promote the kidneys' health and function. A diet rich in fruits and vegetables can help enhance kidney health and prevent kidney disease by supplying necessary nutrients, eliminating pollutants, lowering oxidative stress, and controlling blood sugar levels.

Juicing for Kidney Health

Maintaining a balanced diet.

A well-balanced diet rich in whole fruits and vegetables, lean protein, and whole grains is critical for overall health and the prevention of chronic diseases. Here are some of the primary advantages of eating a well-balanced diet:

It provides the body with the necessary nutrients, vitamins, and minerals that are required for maximum health. Fruits and vegetables are abundant in vitamins and minerals, such as vitamins C and K, potassium, and magnesium, which are necessary for a healthy immune system, strong bones, and the prevention of chronic diseases.

Reducing the Risk of Chronic Diseases: A diet high in fruits and vegetables has been found to lower the risk of chronic diseases such as heart disease, stroke, and some types of cancer. A diet rich in lean protein, such as fish and poultry, and whole grains, such as brown rice and whole wheat, can also help lower the risk of chronic diseases by supplying the body with important nutrients and lowering inflammation.

Maintaining a Healthy Weight: A well-balanced diet rich in whole fruits and vegetables, lean protein, and whole grains can help you maintain a healthy weight by providing your body with critical nutrients and lowering your risk of overeating and weight gain. Furthermore, a fiber-rich diet, such as that found in whole grains and fruits and vegetables, can help to control digestion and lower the risk of obesity.

Improving Brain Health: It has been established that a balanced diet rich in whole fruits and vegetables, lean protein, and whole grains improves brain health and lowers the risk of cognitive decline and dementia. This is because a diet high in minerals and antioxidants can help prevent inflammation and oxidative stress, both of which can contribute to brain health decline.

It includes a range of whole fruits and vegetables, lean protein, and whole grains can assist in maintaining heart health by lowering the risk of heart disease. This is because a diet high in minerals and antioxidants, such as those found in fruits and vegetables, can help lower inflammation and oxidative stress, both of which can contribute to heart disease.

A well-balanced diet rich in whole fruits and vegetables, lean protein, and whole grains is critical for overall health and lowering the risk of chronic diseases. A balanced diet can help promote

Juicing for Kidney Health

optimal health and avoid chronic diseases by providing the body with needed nutrients and lowering inflammation and oxidative stress.

Benefits of juicing for those with chronic kidney disease.

For good reason, juicing has become a trendy practice in recent years. Juicing has numerous potential benefits for those with chronic kidney disease (CKD), including decreased creatinine levels and overall wellness. Here's a closer look at how juicing can benefit people with CKD:

Improved Creatinine Levels: Creatinine is a waste product produced by the muscles and excreted by the kidneys. The kidneys may not operate correctly in people with CKD, resulting in increased creatinine levels in the blood. Juicing can help lower creatinine levels by giving the body antioxidants and anti-inflammatory substances, which can reduce oxidative stress and inflammation in the kidneys. Furthermore, the hydration qualities of many fruits and vegetables can aid in the removal of pollutants and the reduction of creatinine levels.

Enhanced Overall Health: Juicing can enhance overall health in people with CKD by providing the body with critical nutrients, vitamins, and minerals. Fruits and vegetables are rich in antioxidants, anti-inflammatory chemicals, vitamins, and minerals, all of which can help reduce oxidative stress and inflammation in the body, improving overall health and preventing chronic diseases.

Increased Antioxidant and Anti-Inflammatory Qualities: Juicing can boost the body's antioxidant and anti-inflammatory properties, which can aid in the reduction of oxidative stress and inflammation in the kidneys. This is crucial for people with CKD because oxidative stress and inflammation can lead to disease progression and further kidney damage.

Juicing can assist in improving kidney function by providing the body with important nutrients and decreasing oxidative stress and inflammation in the kidneys. This can help to avoid further kidney damage and delay the progression of CKD. Furthermore, the hydration qualities of many fruits and vegetables can aid in the removal of pollutants and the improvement of renal function.

Reduced Toxins: Juicing can aid in the removal of toxins from the body by delivering hydration and antioxidants that aid in the flushing of toxins and the reduction of oxidative stress and

Juicing for Kidney Health

inflammation in the kidneys. Toxins can contribute to increased kidney damage and the course of the disease, which is critical for patients with CKD.

In conclusion, juicing has the potential to provide several benefits for people with chronic kidney disease, including increased creatinine levels, improved general health, increased antioxidant and anti-inflammatory characteristics, improved renal function, and reduced pollutants. Before beginning a juicing plan, consult with your doctor because certain fruits and vegetables may not be suitable for people with kidney problems.

Consult a healthcare provider or registered dietitian.

Before introducing juicing into your diet, talk with a healthcare physician or trained nutritionist. This is especially true for people who have chronic kidney illnesses, as certain fruits and vegetables may not be suitable for them. Here are some of the reasons why you should consult with a healthcare practitioner before beginning a juicing regimen:

Medical Considerations: Before beginning a juicing regimen, address any medical issues or drugs you are taking with your healthcare provider. Specific fruits and vegetables may interact with drugs or be harmful to people with certain medical problems. Your doctor can advise you on which fruits and vegetables are best for your condition.

Nutritional Considerations: A qualified dietitian can assist you in determining the proper nutrient balance in your juicing regimen. They can assist you in determining the best combination of fruits and vegetables to match your specific nutritional needs and ensure that you are getting enough of the vitamins, minerals, and nutrients your body requires to maintain maximum health.

Considerations for Safety: Certain fruits and vegetables have high quantities of oxalates or potassium, which can be detrimental to people who have kidney disease. A healthcare physician or certified nutritionist can advise you on which fruits and vegetables to avoid and suggest alternate options for juicing.

Juicing can be a terrific method to incorporate more fruits and veggies into your diet, but it's vital to keep track of portion amounts. Overconsumption of some fruits and vegetables can cause

Juicing for Kidney Health

dietary imbalances and potential health problems. A licensed dietician can assist you in determining proper portion sizes based on your specific needs and goals.

Personalized Suggestions: A healthcare physician or qualified dietician can make recommendations based on your specific requirements and goals. They can build a juicing routine that is tailored to your medical history, current health status, and personal preferences.

Finally, before beginning a juicing regimen, it is critical to contact a healthcare physician or qualified nutritionist. They can assist you in determining the best combination of fruits and vegetables to match your specific nutritional needs and ensure that you are getting enough of the vitamins, minerals, and nutrients your body requires to maintain maximum health. They can also advise you on any medical or safety concerns, as well as make unique recommendations based on your specific needs and goals.

Incorporating other healthy lifestyle changes.

Incorporating healthy lifestyle changes in addition to juicing can have a substantial influence on overall health and well-being, particularly for those suffering from chronic kidney disease. Here are a few important advantages to making other healthy lifestyle changes:

Excess salt in the diet can cause fluid buildup, elevated blood pressure, and greater strain on the kidneys. Reduced salt consumption can help lower blood pressure and lower the risk of kidney injury. This can be accomplished by lowering the amount of salt added to meals and shopping for low-sodium choices.

Quitting smoking: Smoking is a big risk factor for many health issues, including kidney disease. Quitting smoking can help to lower blood pressure, reduce the risk of kidney damage, and improve general health.

Regular Physical Activity: Exercising on a regular basis can enhance general health and well-being, reduce stress, and help maintain a healthy weight. It can also help with blood pressure and kidney function. Aim for at least 30 minutes of physical activity per day.

Juicing for Kidney Health

Maintaining a Healthy Weight: Being overweight or obese increases the risk of renal disease. Maintaining a healthy weight can help relieve kidney strain and lessen the risk of kidney injury. This can be accomplished by combining healthy eating habits with regular physical activity.

Stress Reduction: Chronic stress can have a negative impact on one's entire health and well-being. It can raise blood pressure and cause the release of toxic hormones, both of which can cause kidney injury. Stress-reduction strategies like meditation, deep breathing, and yoga can help reduce stress and enhance overall health.

Getting Enough Sleep: Adequate sleep is critical for general health and well-being. Adequate sleep can help reduce stress, boost mood, and promote immune system health. Aim for at least 7–8 hours of sleep per night.

Impact of juicing on overall health and well-being.

Juicing is the process of extracting the juice from fruits and vegetables while discarding the pulp and peel in order to receive a concentrated amount of vitamins, minerals, and antioxidants. While there are numerous possible health benefits to juicing, it is critical to recognize the influence it might have on your overall health and well-being.

Enhanced Energy

One of the most frequently mentioned advantages of juicing is an improvement in energy levels. This is partly because fruits and vegetables include high levels of vitamins, minerals, and antioxidants, which can help enhance your immune system, increase your metabolism, and provide a natural source of energy. Juice has a concentrated version of vitamins and minerals that are quickly absorbed by the body, offering a rapid burst of energy that can help you feel more alert and focused throughout the day.

Skin Improvement

Juicing, in addition to raising energy levels, can improve the appearance of your skin. Fruits and vegetables contain antioxidants such as vitamins A and C, which are necessary for healthy skin. Antioxidants assist in protecting the skin from free radical damage, which can contribute to

Juicing for Kidney Health

aging indications such as wrinkles, fine lines, and age spots. Juicing can also help boost the hydration levels of your skin, giving it a more youthful, radiant appearance.

Headaches are less severe. Juicing may provide a natural treatment for people who suffer from headaches on a regular basis. Many fruits and vegetables include natural pain relievers like magnesium and potassium, which can aid with headache symptoms. Furthermore, the high antioxidant levels found in fruits and vegetables might aid in reducing inflammation in the body, which can be a cause of headaches. You can potentially lower the frequency and intensity of your headaches by introducing more fruits and vegetables into your diet through juicing.

While juicing has many benefits for overall health and well-being, it is crucial to remember that it is not a miracle cure. Juicing, like any other dietary adjustment, should be combined with a balanced diet, frequent exercise, and a healthy lifestyle to gain the greatest health advantages. Furthermore, it is critical to be aware of the potential hazards of juicing, such as a lack of fiber and a high sugar content in some juices, and to speak with a healthcare expert before making any major dietary changes.

It can promote general health and well-being by increasing energy, improving skin, and decreasing headaches. However, it is critical to understand the potential hazards and to combine them with a well-balanced diet, regular exercise, and a healthy lifestyle.

In essence, incorporating popular juicing ingredients in one's diet has various potential benefits for overall health and well-being, particularly kidney health.

Fruits and vegetables are high in vitamins, minerals, and antioxidants, which can increase immunity and protect against disease. Cranberries, for example, are a natural diuretic that has been demonstrated to help reduce urinary tract infections and kidney stones. Pomegranates have antioxidant and anti-inflammatory qualities that may help protect the kidneys from free radical damage.

Furthermore, integrating leafy greens like spinach and kale into your diet can offer your body high levels of vitamin K and magnesium, both of which are essential for healthy kidney function. Beetroot is another typical juicing component that is high in nitrates and has been shown to increase blood flow to the kidneys as well as assist overall kidney health.

Juicing for Kidney Health

While it is critical to incorporate these foods into your diet, it is also critical to maintain a dedication to a healthy lifestyle. This involves eating a balanced diet, being physically active, maintaining a healthy weight, avoiding bad habits like smoking and excessive alcohol consumption, and staying physically active.

Maintaining a healthy lifestyle and including juice in your diet can aid in maintaining optimal kidney function and preventing the development of chronic kidney disease. Juicing should be done in moderation, and a healthy diet should always include a variety of fruits, vegetables, and complete grains.

A consultation with a healthcare physician or a certified nutritionist can also be beneficial in identifying the best juicing strategy for your specific needs and health status. We can improve our kidney health and overall well-being by incorporating these popular nutrients into our juicing program.

Juicing for Kidney Health

CHAPTER 7

Juice Recipes for Supporting Kidney Health

Emmanuelle was discovered to have a kidney illness. She was devastated by the news and felt helpless to remedy her health. Her doctor, on the other hand, advised her to make some lifestyle modifications, such as introducing more fresh juices into her diet.

Emmanuelle was initially apprehensive but decided to give it a shot. She began researching the finest juice recipes for kidney health and discovered the numerous benefits of including fruits and vegetables in her diet. Certain components, such as cranberries, beets, and lemons, she discovered, might help reduce inflammation and promote detoxification, which was beneficial to her kidneys.

She was motivated to be more creative in the kitchen and began experimenting with various juice concoctions. She discovered that not only were the fresh, handmade juices delightful, but they also offered her a substantial energy boost. She noted that as she continued to add more juices to her diet, her overall health improved and her kidney function stabilized.

Emmanuelle was astounded by the positive changes in her health and thankful to have discovered an easy and pleasurable technique to help her kidneys. She was so enthusiastic about the health advantages of juice that she launched a blog to share her experience and the great juice recipes she had discovered. Her blog immediately grew in popularity, inspiring many others to begin integrating more fresh juices into their diets.

Years later, She is still going strong and sharing her passion for juice and its incredible health advantages. She is delighted to have motivated others to take charge of their health, and she is appreciative for the great influence juice has had on her life.

Juicing for Kidney Health

30 juicing recipes for preventive kidney care.

Carrot, Ginger, and Apple Juice.

Ingredients:

4 large carrots

1 medium-sized ginger root

2 medium-sized apples

1 cup water

Instructions:

Wash the carrots, ginger, and apples thoroughly.

Cut the carrots and apples into small pieces and peel the ginger.

Put the chopped carrots, ginger, apples, and water in a blender.

Blend the ingredients until smooth.

Strain the juice through a fine mesh strainer to remove any remaining pulp.

Pour the juice into a glass and enjoy immediately.

Note: You can adjust the amount of ginger based on your preference. Adding more ginger can make the juice spicier

Cucumber, Lime, and Mint Juice.

Ingredients:

2 medium-sized cucumbers

2 limes, peeled and seeded

Juicing for Kidney Health

1 cup fresh mint leaves

1 cup water

Instructions:

Wash the cucumbers, limes, and mint thoroughly.

Cut the cucumbers into small pieces.

Put the chopped cucumbers, lime segments, mint leaves, and water in a blender.

Blend the ingredients until smooth.

Strain the juice through a fine mesh strainer to remove any remaining pulp.

Pour the juice into a glass and enjoy immediately.

Note: You can adjust the amount of mint leaves based on your preference. Adding more mint can make the juice more flavorful.

Beets, Apples, and Carrots Juice.

Ingredients:

2 medium-sized beets

2 medium-sized apples

4 large carrots

1 cup water

Instructions:

Wash the beets, apples, and carrots thoroughly.

Cut the beets, apples, and carrots into small pieces.

Juicing for Kidney Health

Put the chopped beets, apples, carrots, and water in a blender.

Blend the ingredients until smooth.

Strain the juice through a fine mesh strainer to remove any remaining pulp.

Pour the juice into a glass and enjoy immediately.

Note: You can adjust the amount of ingredients based on your preference. Adding more apples can make the juice sweeter.

Cucumber, Kale, and Spinach Juice.

Ingredients:

2 medium-sized cucumbers

4 cups kale leaves

4 cups spinach leaves

1 cup water

Instructions:

Wash the cucumbers, kale, and spinach thoroughly.

Cut the cucumbers into small pieces.

Put the chopped cucumbers, kale, spinach, and water in a blender.

Blend the ingredients until smooth.

Strain the juice through a fine mesh strainer to remove any remaining pulp.

Pour the juice into a glass and enjoy immediately.

Note: You can adjust the amount of kale and spinach based on your preference. Adding more kale and spinach can make the juice more nutritious

Juicing for Kidney Health

Apple, Cinnamon, and Parsley Juice.

Ingredients:

4 medium-sized apples

1 teaspoon cinnamon powder

1 cup fresh parsley leaves

1 cup water

Instructions:

Wash the apples and parsley thoroughly.

Cut the apples into small pieces.

Put the chopped apples, cinnamon powder, parsley, and water in a blender.

Blend the ingredients until smooth.

Strain the juice through a fine mesh strainer to remove any remaining pulp.

Pour the juice into a glass and enjoy immediately.

Note: You can adjust the amount of cinnamon based on your preference. Adding more cinnamon can make the juice spicier

Carrot, Orange, and Ginger Juice.

Ingredients:

4 large carrots

2 medium-sized oranges, peeled and seeded

1 medium-sized ginger root

1 cup water

Juicing for Kidney Health

Instructions:

Wash the carrots, oranges, and ginger thoroughly.

Cut the carrots into small pieces and peel the ginger.

Put the chopped carrots, orange segments, ginger, and water in a blender.

Blend the ingredients until smooth.

Strain the juice through a fine mesh strainer to remove any remaining pulp.

Pour the juice into a glass and enjoy immediately.

Note: You can adjust the amount of ginger based on your preference. Adding more ginger can make the juice spicier.

Spinach, Apple, and Lemon Juice.

Ingredients:

4 cups spinach leaves

2 medium-sized apples

1 medium-sized lemon, peeled and seeded

1 cup water

Instructions:

Wash the spinach, apples, and lemon thoroughly.

Cut the apples into small pieces.

Put the spinach, chopped apples, lemon segments, and water in a blender.

Blend the ingredients until smooth.

Juicing for Kidney Health

Strain the juice through a fine mesh strainer to remove any remaining pulp.

Pour the juice into a glass and enjoy immediately.

Note: You can adjust the amount of lemon based on your preference. Adding more lemon can make the juice sourer.

Kale, Cucumber, and Pineapple Juice.

Ingredients:

4 cups kale leaves

2 medium-sized cucumbers

2 cups fresh pineapple, peeled and cored

1 cup water

Instructions:

Wash the kale, cucumbers, and pineapple thoroughly.

Cut the cucumbers and pineapple into small pieces.

Put the kale, chopped cucumbers, pineapple, and water in a blender.

Blend the ingredients until smooth.

Strain the juice through a fine mesh strainer to remove any remaining pulp.

Pour the juice into a glass and enjoy immediately.

Note: You can adjust the amount of pineapple based on your preference. Adding more pineapple can make the juice sweeter.

Carrot, Beet, and Apple Juice.

Juicing for Kidney Health

Ingredients:

4 large carrots

2 medium-sized beets

2 medium-sized apples

1 cup water

Instructions:

Wash the carrots, beets, and apples thoroughly.

Cut the carrots and apples into small pieces.

Put the chopped carrots, beets, apples, and water in a blender.

Blend the ingredients until smooth.

Strain the juice through a fine mesh strainer to remove any remaining pulp.

Pour the juice into a glass and enjoy immediately.

Note: You can adjust the amount of beets based on your preference. Adding more beets can make the juice earthier.

Cucumber, Spinach, and Ginger Juice.

Ingredients:

2 medium-sized cucumbers

4 cups spinach leaves

1 medium-sized ginger root

1 cup water

Juicing for Kidney Health

Instructions:

Wash the cucumbers, spinach, and ginger thoroughly.

Cut the cucumbers into small pieces and peel the ginger.

Put the chopped cucumbers, spinach, ginger, and water in a blender.

Blend the ingredients until smooth.

Strain the juice through a fine mesh strainer to remove any remaining pulp.

Pour the juice into a glass and enjoy immediately.

Note: You can adjust the amount of ginger based on your preference. Adding more ginger can make the juice spicier.

Pineapple, Mint, and Lime Juice.

Ingredients:

2 cups fresh pineapple, peeled and cored

1 cup fresh mint leaves

1 medium-sized lime, peeled and seeded

1 cup water

Instructions:

Wash the pineapple, mint, and lime thoroughly.

Cut the pineapple into small pieces.

Put the pineapple, mint leaves, lime segments, and water in a blender.

Juicing for Kidney Health

Blend the ingredients until smooth.

Strain the juice through a fine mesh strainer to remove any remaining pulp.

Pour the juice into a glass and enjoy immediately.

Note: You can adjust the amount of lime based on your preference. Adding more lime can make the juice sourer.

Apple, Ginger, and Parsley Juice.

Ingredients:

4 medium-sized apples

1 medium-sized ginger root

1 cup fresh parsley leaves

1 cup water

Instructions:

Wash the apples, ginger, and parsley thoroughly.

Cut the apples into small pieces and peel the ginger.

Put the chopped apples, ginger, parsley, and water in a blender.

Blend the ingredients until smooth.

Strain the juice through a fine mesh strainer to remove any remaining pulp.

Pour the juice into a glass and enjoy immediately.

Note: You can adjust the amount of ginger based on your preference. Adding more ginger can make the juice spicier.

Carrot, Cucumber, and Celery Juice.

Juicing for Kidney Health

Ingredients:

4 large carrots

2 medium-sized cucumbers

4 stalks of celery

1 cup water

Instructions:

Wash the carrots, cucumbers, and celery thoroughly.

Cut the carrots and celery into small pieces.

Put the chopped carrots, cucumbers, celery, and water in a blender.

Blend the ingredients until smooth.

Strain the juice through a fine mesh strainer to remove any remaining pulp.

Pour the juice into a glass and enjoy immediately.

Note: You can adjust the amount of celery based on your preference. Adding more celery can make the juice savorier.

Kale, Spinach, and Pear Juice.

Ingredients:

4 cups kale leaves

4 cups spinach leaves

2 medium-sized pears

1 cup water

Juicing for Kidney Health

Instructions:

Wash the kale, spinach, and pears thoroughly.

Cut the pears into small pieces.

Put the kale, spinach, pears, and water in a blender.

Blend the ingredients until smooth.

Strain the juice through a fine mesh strainer to remove any remaining pulp.

Pour the juice into a glass and enjoy immediately.

Note: You can adjust the amount of pears based on your preference.

Carrot, Apple, and Lemon Juice.

Ingredients:

4 large carrots

2 medium-sized apples

1 medium-sized lemon, peeled and seeded

1 cup water

Instructions:

Wash the carrots, apples, and lemon thoroughly.

Cut the carrots and apples into small pieces.

Put the chopped carrots, apples, lemon segments, and water in a blender.

Blend the ingredients until smooth.

Strain the juice through a fine mesh strainer to remove any remaining pulp.

Pour the juice into a glass and enjoy immediately.

Juicing for Kidney Health

Note: You can adjust the amount of lemon based on your preference. Adding more lemon can make the juice sourer.

Cucumber, Grapefruit, and Ginger Juice.

Ingredients:

2 medium-sized cucumbers

1 medium-sized grapefruit, peeled and seeded

1 inch piece of ginger root

1 cup water

Instructions:

Wash the cucumbers, grapefruit, and ginger thoroughly.

Cut the cucumbers and grapefruit into small pieces.

Peel the ginger and cut it into small pieces.

Put the chopped cucumbers, grapefruit, ginger, and water in a blender.

Blend the ingredients until smooth.

Strain the juice through a fine mesh strainer to remove any remaining pulp.

Pour the juice into a glass and enjoy immediately.

Note: You can adjust the amount of ginger based on your preference. More ginger can make the juice spicier.

Beets, Carrots, and Ginger Juice.

Ingredients:

Juicing for Kidney Health

2 medium-sized beets

4 large carrots

1 inch piece of ginger root

1 cup water

Instructions:

Wash the beets, carrots, and ginger thoroughly.

Cut the beets and carrots into small pieces.

Peel the ginger and cut it into small pieces.

Put the chopped beets, carrots, ginger, and water in a blender.

Blend the ingredients until smooth.

Strain the juice through a fine mesh strainer to remove any remaining pulp.

Pour the juice into a glass and enjoy immediately.

Note: You can adjust the amount of ginger based on your preference. Adding more ginger can make the juice spicier.

Spinach, Cucumber, and Lemon Juice.

Ingredients:

4 cups spinach leaves

2 medium-sized cucumbers

1 medium-sized lemon, peeled and seeded

1 cup water

Juicing for Kidney Health

Instructions:

Wash the spinach, cucumbers, and lemon thoroughly.

Cut the cucumbers and lemon into small pieces.

Put the spinach, cucumbers, lemon segments, and water in a blender.

Blend the ingredients until smooth.

Strain the juice through a fine mesh strainer to remove any remaining pulp.

Pour the juice into a glass and enjoy immediately.

Note: You can adjust the amount of lemon based on your preference. Adding more lemon can make the juice sourer.

Apple, Carrot, and Celery Juice.

Ingredients:

2 medium-sized apples

4 large carrots

4 celery stalks

1 cup water

Instructions:

Wash the apples, carrots, and celery thoroughly.

Cut the apples and carrots into small pieces.

Cut the celery stalks into small pieces.

Put the chopped apples, carrots, celery, and water in a blender.

Blend the ingredients until smooth.

Juicing for Kidney Health

Strain the juice through a fine mesh strainer to remove any remaining pulp.

Pour the juice into a glass and enjoy immediately

Cucumber, Mint, and Grapefruit Juice.

Ingredients:

2 medium-sized cucumbers

1 medium-sized grapefruit, peeled and seeded

1/2 cup fresh mint leaves

1 cup water

Instructions:

Wash the cucumbers, grapefruit, and mint thoroughly.

Cut the cucumbers and grapefruit into small pieces.

Put the chopped cucumbers, grapefruit, mint leaves, and water in a blender.

Blend the ingredients until smooth.

Strain the juice through a fine mesh strainer to remove any remaining pulp.

Pour the juice into a glass and enjoy immediately

Carrot, Orange, and Turmeric Juice.

Ingredients:

4 large carrots

2 medium-sized oranges, peeled and seeded

1 inch piece of fresh turmeric root or 1/2 teaspoon ground turmeric

Juicing for Kidney Health

1 cup water

Instructions:

Wash the carrots, oranges, and turmeric thoroughly.

Cut the carrots into small pieces.

Peel the turmeric and cut it into small pieces (if using fresh turmeric).

Put the chopped carrots, oranges, turmeric, and water in a blender.

Blend the ingredients until smooth.

Strain the juice through a fine mesh strainer to remove any remaining pulp.

Pour the juice into a glass and enjoy immediately.

Spinach, Kale, and Apple Juice.

Ingredients:

2 cups packed spinach leaves

2 cups packed kale leaves

2 medium-sized apples

1 cup water

Instructions:

Wash the spinach, kale, and apples thoroughly.

Cut the apples into small pieces.

Put the packed spinach, kale, chopped apples, and water in a blender.

Blend the ingredients until smooth.

Juicing for Kidney Health

Strain the juice through a fine mesh strainer to remove any remaining pulp.

Pour the juice into a glass and enjoy immediately.

Carrot, Beet, and Ginger Juice.

Ingredients:

4 large carrots

2 medium-sized beets

1 inch piece of fresh ginger root

1 cup water

Instructions:

Wash the carrots, beets, and ginger thoroughly.

Cut the carrots and beets into small pieces.

Peel the ginger and cut it into small pieces.

Put the chopped carrots, beets, ginger, and water in a blender.

Blend the ingredients until smooth.

Strain the juice through a fine mesh strainer to remove any remaining pulp.

Pour the juice into a glass and drink immediately

Cucumber, Pear, and Ginger Juice.

Ingredients:

Juicing for Kidney Health

2 medium-sized cucumbers

2 medium-sized pears

1 inch piece of fresh ginger root

1 cup water

Instructions:

Wash the cucumbers, pears, and ginger thoroughly.

Cut the cucumbers and pears into small pieces.

Peel the ginger and cut it into small pieces.

Put the chopped cucumbers, pears, ginger, and water in a blender.

Blend the ingredients until smooth.

Strain the juice through a fine mesh strainer to remove any remaining pulp.

Pour the juice into a glass and enjoy immediately

Apple, Cinnamon, and Carrot Juice.

Ingredients:

4 medium-sized apples

2 large carrots

1 teaspoon ground cinnamon

1 cup water

Instructions:

Wash the apples and carrots thoroughly.

Juicing for Kidney Health

Cut the apples and carrots into small pieces.

Put the chopped apples, carrots, cinnamon, and water in a blender.

Blend the ingredients until smooth.

Strain the juice through a fine mesh strainer to remove any remaining pulp.

Pour the juice into a glass and drink immediately

Spinach, Cucumber, and Apple Juice.

Ingredients:

2 cups packed spinach leaves

2 medium-sized cucumbers

2 medium-sized apples

1 cup water

Instructions:

Wash the spinach, cucumbers, and apples thoroughly.

Cut the cucumbers and apples into small pieces.

Put the spinach, chopped cucumbers, apples, and water in a blender.

Blend the ingredients until smooth.

Strain the juice through a fine mesh strainer to remove any remaining pulp.

Pour the juice into a glass and enjoy immediately

Carrot, Grapefruit, and Ginger Juice.

Ingredients:

Juicing for Kidney Health

4 large carrots

1 medium-sized grapefruit, peeled and seeded

1 medium-sized ginger root

1 cup water

Instructions:

Wash the carrots, grapefruit, and ginger thoroughly.

Cut the carrots into small pieces and peel the ginger.

Put the chopped carrots, grapefruit segments, ginger, and water in a blender.

Blend the ingredients until smooth.

Strain the juice through a fine mesh strainer to remove any remaining pulp.

Pour the juice into a glass and drink immediately.

Note: You can adjust the amount of ginger based on your preference. Adding more ginger can make the juice spicier.

Cucumber, Kale, and Apple Juice.

Ingredients:

2 medium-sized cucumbers

2 cups packed kale leaves

2 medium-sized apples

1 cup water

Instructions:

Wash the cucumbers, kale, and apples thoroughly.

Juicing for Kidney Health

Cut the cucumbers and apples into small pieces.

Put the chopped cucumbers, kale, apples, and water in a blender.

Blend the ingredients until smooth.

Strain the juice through a fine mesh strainer to remove any remaining pulp.

Pour the juice into a glass and drink immediately

Beets, Carrots, and Apple Juice.

Ingredients:

2 medium-sized beets

4 medium-sized carrots

2 medium-sized apples

1 cup water

Instructions:

Wash the beets, carrots, and apples thoroughly.

Cut the beets and carrots into small pieces.

Peel and core the apples, and cut them into small pieces.

Put the chopped beets, carrots, apples, and water in a blender.

Blend the ingredients until smooth.

Strain the juice through a fine mesh strainer to remove any remaining pulp.

Pour the juice into a glass and drink immediately.

Spinach, Pear, and Ginger Juice.

Juicing for Kidney Health

Ingredients:

4 cups packed spinach leaves

2 medium-sized pears

1-inch piece of ginger root

1 cup water

Instructions:

Wash the spinach, pears, and ginger thoroughly.

Cut the pears into small pieces and peel the ginger root.

Put the packed spinach leaves, chopped pears, ginger, and water in a blender.

Blend the ingredients until smooth.

Strain the juice through a fine mesh strainer to remove any remaining pulp.

Pour the juice into a glass and drink immediately.

20 RECIPES FOR THOSE WITH MILD KIDNEY DISEASE.

Cucumber, Kale, and Apple Juice:

Ingredients:

4 cups kale

2 medium-sized cucumbers

2 medium-sized apples

1 cup water

Juicing for Kidney Health

Instructions:

Wash the kale, cucumbers, and apples thoroughly.

Cut the cucumbers and apples into small pieces.

Put the kale, cucumbers, apples, and water in a blender.

Blend the ingredients until smooth.

Strain the juice through a fine mesh strainer to remove any remaining pulp.

Pour the juice into a glass and drink instantly.

Carrot, Apple, and Ginger Juice:

Ingredients:

6 medium-sized carrots

2 medium-sized apples

1-inch piece of ginger root

1 cup water

Instructions:

Wash the carrots, apples, and ginger root thoroughly.

Cut the carrots and apples into small pieces.

Peel the ginger root.

Put the chopped carrots, apples, ginger root, and water in a blender.

Blend the ingredients until smooth.

Strain the juice through a fine mesh strainer to remove any remaining pulp.

Pour the juice into a glass and enjoy immediately.

Juicing for Kidney Health

Spinach, Cucumber, and Lemon Juice.

Ingredients:

4 cups packed spinach leaves

2 medium-sized cucumbers

1 medium-sized lemon

1 cup water

Instructions:

Wash the spinach, cucumbers, and lemon thoroughly.

Cut the cucumbers into small pieces.

Squeeze the lemon to extract the juice.

Put the packed spinach leaves, chopped cucumbers, lemon juice, and water in a blender.

Blend the ingredients until smooth.

Strain the juice through a fine mesh strainer to remove any remaining pulp.

Pour the juice into a glass and enjoy immediately.

Carrot, Orange, and Ginger Juice:

Ingredients:

6 medium-sized carrots

2 medium-sized oranges

1-inch piece of ginger root

1 cup water

Juicing for Kidney Health

Instructions:

Wash the carrots, oranges, and ginger root thoroughly.

Cut the carrots into small pieces.

Peel the oranges and ginger root.

Put the chopped carrots, oranges, ginger root, and water in a blender.

Blend the ingredients until smooth.

Strain the juice through a fine mesh strainer to remove any remaining pulp.

Pour the juice into a glass and drink immediately

Apple, Cinnamon, and Parsley Juice:

Ingredients:

4 medium-sized apples

1 teaspoon of ground cinnamon

1 handful of parsley leaves

1 cup water

Instructions:

Wash the apples and parsley thoroughly.

Core the apples and cut them into small pieces.

Put the chopped apples, ground cinnamon, parsley, and water in a blender.

Blend the ingredients until smooth.

Strain the juice through a fine mesh strainer to remove any remaining pulp.

Juicing for Kidney Health

Drink immediately.

Cucumber, Spinach, and Ginger Juice:

Ingredients:

2 medium-sized cucumbers

4 cups packed spinach leaves

1-inch piece of ginger root

1 cup water

Instructions:

Wash the cucumbers, spinach, and ginger thoroughly.

Cut the cucumbers into small pieces and peel the ginger root.

Put the chopped cucumbers, packed spinach leaves, ginger, and water in a blender.

Blend the ingredients until smooth.

Strain the juice through a fine mesh strainer to remove any remaining pulp.

Pour the juice into a glass and enjoy immediately.

Carrot, Apple, and Celery Juice:

Ingredients:

4 medium-sized carrots

4 medium-sized apples

4 celery stalks

1 cup water

Juicing for Kidney Health

Instructions:

Wash the carrots, apples, and celery thoroughly.

Cut the carrots and celery into small pieces.

Peel and core the apples and cut them into small pieces.

Put the chopped carrots, apples, celery, and water in a blender.

Blend the ingredients until smooth.

Strain the juice through a fine mesh strainer to remove any remaining pulp.

Pour the juice into a glass and enjoy immediately.

Kale, Cucumber, and Pineapple Juice:

Ingredients:

4 cups packed kale leaves

2 medium-sized cucumbers

2 cups fresh pineapple chunks

1 cup water

Instructions:

Wash the kale, cucumbers, and pineapple thoroughly.

Cut the cucumbers into small pieces and chop the kale leaves.

Cut the pineapple into small pieces.

Put the chopped kale, cucumbers, pineapple, and water in a blender.

Blend the ingredients until smooth.

Juicing for Kidney Health

Strain the juice through a fine mesh strainer to remove any remaining pulp.

Pour the juice into a glass and enjoy immediately.

Beets, Carrots, and Apple Juice.

Ingredients:

2 medium-sized beets, peeled and chopped

3 large carrots, peeled and chopped

2 medium-sized apples, cored and chopped

Instructions:

Wash the beets, carrots, and apples thoroughly.

Chop the beets, carrots, and apples into small pieces.

Run the chopped vegetables and fruit through a juicer and collect the juice in a glass.

Stir the juice well to combine.

Serve the juice immediately and enjoy!

Note: You can add some ginger to the juice for added flavor and health benefits

Carrot, Beet, and Ginger Juice.

Ingredients:

2 medium beets, peeled and chopped

4 large carrots, peeled and chopped

1 inch piece of ginger, peeled and chopped

2 medium apples, cored and chopped

Juicing for Kidney Health

filtered water (if needed)

Instructions:

Rinse and chop the beets, carrots, ginger, and apples into small pieces that can fit in your juicer.

Pass the chopped vegetables and fruit through your juicer, following the manufacturer's instructions.

If the juice is too thick, add some filtered water to thin it out to your desired consistency.

Serve the juice immediately, or store it in an airtight glass container in the refrigerator for up to 24 hours.

Enjoy your delicious and healthy Juice.

Cucumber, Grapefruit, and Ginger Juice.

Cucumber, Grapefruit, and Ginger Juice Recipe:

Ingredients:

2 medium sized cucumbers

2 medium sized grapefruits

1-2 inch piece of ginger

1/4 teaspoon salt (optional)

Instructions:

Wash and peel the cucumbers, grapefruits, and ginger.

Cut the grapefruits into segments and remove the seeds.

Cut the cucumbers and ginger into small pieces.

Juicing for Kidney Health

Put the grapefruit segments, cucumber pieces, and ginger into a juicer and juice until smooth.

Stir in the salt (if using).

Pour the juice into a glass and serve immediately. Enjoy

Apple, Cinnamon, and Carrot Juice

Ingredients:

3 medium-sized apples

2 medium-sized carrots

1 teaspoon of cinnamon

1/4 cup of water (optional)

Instructions:

Wash and chop the apples and carrots into small pieces.

Put the chopped apples and carrots in a juicer.

Add cinnamon to the juicer.

If desired, add 1/4 cup of water to the juicer to thin the juice.

Start the juicer and let it run until all the ingredients have been juiced.

Pour the juice into a glass and enjoy immediately.

This Apple, Cinnamon, and Carrot juice is a sweet and delicious way to boost your energy and support your kidney health. The carrots and apples are rich in antioxidants and vitamins that help prevent oxidative stress and inflammation, while the cinnamon adds a warming and flavorful touch

Carrot, Orange, and Turmeric Juice.

Juicing for Kidney Health

Ingredients:

4 medium carrots, washed and chopped

2 medium oranges, peeled

1 inch piece of fresh turmeric root, peeled

1 tsp honey (optional)

Instructions:

Wash and chop the carrots and set aside.

Peel the oranges and set aside.

Peel the turmeric root and set aside.

Add the carrots, oranges, and turmeric root to a juicer and juice until smooth.

If desired, add 1 tsp of honey to the juice and stir to combine.

Pour the juice into a glass and drink immediately

Cucumber, Pear, and Ginger Juice.

Ingredients:

2 medium cucumbers

2 medium pears

1 inch piece of ginger

Instructions:

Wash and peel the cucumbers and pears, removing any seeds if necessary.

Cut the ginger into small pieces.

Juicing for Kidney Health

Run all the ingredients through a juicer and collect the juice in a glass.

Stir the juice well and serve immediately, garnished with a slice of pear or cucumber if desired.

Enjoy your Juice.

Spinach, Cucumber, and Lemon Juice.

Ingredients:

2 cups of fresh spinach

1 large cucumber

1 medium-sized lemon

Water as needed

Instructions:

Wash the spinach, cucumber, and lemon thoroughly.

Cut the lemon into halves, remove the seeds and any white pith.

Cut the cucumber into smaller pieces to fit into the juicer chute.

Put the spinach, cucumber, and lemon halves into the juicer.

Turn on the juicer and juice the ingredients until smooth.

If the juice is too thick, add water as needed to dilute.

Pour the juice into a glass, stir and enjoy immediately.

Note: You can adjust the quantity of the ingredients based on your preference.

Beets, Carrots, and Ginger Juice.

Juicing for Kidney Health

Ingredients:

3 medium-sized beets, peeled and chopped

4 medium-sized carrots, peeled and chopped

1-inch piece of fresh ginger, peeled

1 lemon, juiced

2 cups water

Instructions:

Wash and prepare all the ingredients.

Add the beets, carrots, and ginger to a juicer.

Add lemon juice and 2 cups of water to the juicer.

Juice everything together until you have a smooth mixture.

Strain the juice to remove any remaining pulp or seeds.

Serve immediately and enjoy the health benefits of the juice.

Carrot, Apple, and Lemon Juice.

Ingredients:

2 medium sized carrots

2 medium sized apples

1 lemon, peeled

Water (as required)

Instructions:

Juicing for Kidney Health

Wash and peel the carrots and apples.

Cut the lemon in half and remove the seeds.

Cut the apples into wedges and the carrots into small pieces.

Add the carrots, apples, and lemon to a juicer and process until smooth.

Pour the juice into a glass and add water to taste, if desired.

Stir the juice and serve immediately.

Enjoy your healthy and delicious Carrot, Apple, and Lemon Juice!

Apple, Ginger, and Parsley Juice.

Ingredients:

2 medium apples, cored and chopped

1 inch of fresh ginger root, peeled

1 cup of fresh parsley leaves

1/2 lemon, juiced

Instructions:

Wash the apples, ginger root, and parsley thoroughly.

Chop the apples into small pieces.

Peel the ginger root and chop it into small pieces.

Remove the stems from the parsley leaves.

Put all ingredients into a juicer and extract the juice.

Pour the juice into a glass and add the lemon juice.

Stir well and serve immediately.

Juicing for Kidney Health

Enjoy the fresh and healthy juice!

Cucumber, Mint, and Grapefruit Juice.

Ingredients:

2 medium sized cucumbers

1 medium sized grapefruit

1 cup of fresh mint leaves

1 tsp honey (optional)

1/4 cup of water

Ice (optional)

Instructions:

Wash and peel the cucumbers, grapefruit and remove the mint leaves from their stems.

Cut the cucumbers, grapefruit, and mint into small pieces that can easily fit into a blender.

Add the cucumber, grapefruit, mint, honey (if using), and water to a blender and blend until smooth.

If you prefer, you can strain the juice to remove any pulp or seeds.

Add ice to the blender and pulse until combined, or add to glasses with ice.

Serve immediately and enjoy.

Carrot, Cucumber, and Celery Juice.

Ingredients:

4 medium sized carrots

Juicing for Kidney Health

2 medium sized cucumbers

4 stalks of celery

1 lemon, peeled

1 inch of ginger, peeled (optional)

1/4 cup of water

Ice (optional)

Instructions:

Wash and peel the carrots, cucumbers, and ginger (if using).

Cut the carrots, cucumbers, celery, lemon, and ginger (if using) into small pieces that can easily fit into a blender.

Add the carrots, cucumbers, celery, lemon, ginger (if using), and water to a blender and blend until smooth.

If you prefer, you can strain the juice to remove any pulp or seeds.

Add ice to the blender and pulse until combined, or add to glasses with ice.

Serve immediately and enjoy

Kale, Spinach, and Pear Juice.

Ingredients:

4 cups of kale leaves

2 cups of spinach

2 medium sized pears

1 lemon, peeled

Juicing for Kidney Health

1 inch of ginger, peeled (optional)

1/4 cup of water

Ice (optional)

Instructions:

Wash and stem the kale and spinach.

Peel and core the pears.

Cut the pears, lemon, and ginger (if using) into small pieces that can easily fit into a blender.

Add the kale, spinach, pears, lemon, ginger (if using), and water to a blender and blend until smooth.

If you prefer, you can strain the juice to remove any pulp or seeds.

Add ice to the blender and pulse until combined, or add to glasses with ice.

Serve immediately and enjoy.

20 RECIPES FOR THOSE WITH ADVANCED KIDNEY DISEASE.

Low-Potassium Carrot and Apple Juice.

Ingredients:

3 medium-sized carrots

2 medium-sized apples

1 lemon, peeled and seeded

1 inch of ginger

1 cup of water

Juicing for Kidney Health

Instructions:

Wash and peel the carrots, apples, lemon and ginger.

Cut the ingredients into small pieces that can easily fit into a juicer.

Put the carrot pieces into the juicer, followed by the apples, lemon, and ginger.

Add 1 cup of water to the juicer and blend until everything is well combined.

Strain the juice through a fine mesh strainer to remove any solids.

Serve immediately and enjoy!

Note: Apples are naturally low in potassium, but if you want to lower the potassium levels further, consider using green apples instead of red apples. Additionally, adding water can dilute the juice and reduce the potassium levels.

Cucumber, Lime, and Ginger Juice.

Ingredients:

2 medium-sized cucumbers

2 medium-sized limes

1 inch of ginger root

1 cup of water (optional)

Instructions:

Wash and peel the cucumbers, limes, and ginger root.

Cut the ingredients into small pieces that can easily fit into a juicer.

Put the cucumber pieces into the juicer, followed by the limes and ginger.

If desired, add 1 cup of water to the juicer to help the ingredients blend more easily.

Juicing for Kidney Health

Blend the ingredients until they are well combined.

Strain the juice through a fine mesh strainer to remove any solids.

Serve the juice immediately, over ice if desired.

Enjoy your refreshing and healthy Cucumber, Lime, and Ginger Juice! The cucumber provides hydration and the lime adds a burst of citrus flavor, while the ginger adds a subtle spiciness. This juice is a great way to start your day or to cool down on a hot summer day.

Lightly Steamed Broccoli and Cucumber Juice.

Ingredients:

2 medium-sized broccoli florets

1 medium-sized cucumber

1 lemon, peeled and seeded

1 cup of water (optional)

Instructions:

Wash the broccoli florets, cucumber, and lemon.

Cut the ingredients into small pieces that can easily fit into a juicer.

Lightly steam the broccoli florets for 2-3 minutes to make them easier to blend.

Put the broccoli florets and cucumber into the juicer, followed by the lemon.

If desired, add 1 cup of water to the juicer to help the ingredients blend more easily.

Blend the ingredients until they are well combined.

Strain the juice through a fine mesh strainer to remove any solids.

Serve the juice immediately, over ice if desired.

Juicing for Kidney Health

This Lightly Steamed Broccoli and Cucumber Juice is a nutritious and delicious way to get your daily dose of greens. The lightly steaming of the broccoli helps to preserve its nutrients, while the cucumber and lemon provide a light and refreshing taste

Carrot, Celery, and Lemon Juice.

Ingredients:

4 medium-sized carrots

4 stalks of celery

1 lemon, peeled and seeded

1 cup of water (optional)

Instructions:

Wash the carrots, celery, and lemon.

Cut the ingredients into small pieces that can easily fit into a juicer.

Put the carrot pieces into the juicer, followed by the celery and lemon.

If desired, add 1 cup of water to the juicer to help the ingredients blend more easily.

Blend the ingredients until they are well combined.

Strain the juice through a fine mesh strainer to remove any solids.

Serve the juice immediately, over ice if desired.

The Carrot, Celery, and Lemon Juice is a nutritious and tasty way to start your day or to refresh yourself after a workout. The carrots provide beta-carotene and other vitamins and minerals, while the celery and lemon add a fresh, light flavor to the juice.

Juicing for Kidney Health

Apple, Pear, and Cinnamon Juice.

Ingredients:

2 medium-sized apples

2 medium-sized pears

1 teaspoon of ground cinnamon

1 cup of water (optional)

Instructions:

Wash the apples and pears.

Cut the apples and pears into small pieces that can easily fit into a juicer.

Put the apple and pear pieces into the juicer.

If desired, add 1 cup of water to the juicer to help the ingredients blend more easily.

Sprinkle the ground cinnamon over the top of the ingredients in the juicer.

Blend the ingredients until they are well combined.

Strain the juice through a fine mesh strainer to remove any solids.

Serve the juice immediately with ice if desired.

Apple, Pear, and Cinnamon Juice is a sweet and nutritious way to start your day or to refresh yourself after a workout. Apples and pears provide natural sweetness and vitamins, while the cinnamon adds a warm and spicy flavor to the juice.

Cucumber, Ginger, and Mint Juice.

Ingredients:

2 medium-sized cucumbers

1 inch of ginger root

Juicing for Kidney Health

1 cup of fresh mint leaves

1 cup of water (optional)

Instructions:

Wash the cucumbers, ginger root, and mint leaves.

Cut the cucumbers and ginger root into small pieces that can easily fit into a juicer.

Put the cucumber pieces into the juicer, followed by the ginger and mint leaves.

If desired, add 1 cup of water to the juicer to help the ingredients blend more easily.

Blend the ingredients until they are well combined.

Strain the juice through a fine mesh strainer to remove any solids.

Serve the juice immediately, over ice if desired.

This Cucumber, Ginger, and Mint Juice is a refreshing and healthy way to start your day or to cool down on a hot summer day. The cucumber provides hydration, while the ginger adds a subtle spiciness and the mint adds a burst of fresh flavor to the juice. Enjoy.

Orange and Ginger Juice.

Ingredients:

4 medium-sized oranges

1 inch of ginger root

1 cup of water (optional)

Instructions:

Wash the oranges and ginger root.

Juicing for Kidney Health

Cut the oranges in half and remove the peel, being careful to remove as much of the white pith as possible.

Cut the ginger root into small pieces that can easily fit into a juicer.

Put the orange halves into the juicer, followed by the ginger pieces.

If desired, add 1 cup of water to the juicer to help the ingredients blend more easily.

Blend the ingredients until they are well combined.

Strain the juice through a fine mesh strainer to remove any solids.

Serve the juice immediately, over ice if desired.

Orange and Ginger Juice is a sweet and healthy way to start your day or to refresh yourself. Oranges provide natural sweetness and Vitamin C, while the ginger adds a subtle spiciness to the juice.

Carrot, Blueberry, and Grape Juice.

Ingredients:

4 medium-sized carrots

1 cup of blueberries

1 cup of grapes

1 cup of water (optional)

Instructions:

Wash the carrots, blueberries, and grapes.

Cut the carrots into small pieces that can easily fit into a juicer.

Put the carrot pieces into the juicer, followed by the blueberries and grapes.

If desired, add 1 cup of water to the juicer to help the ingredients blend more easily.

Juicing for Kidney Health

Blend the ingredients until they are well combined.

Strain the juice through a fine mesh strainer to remove any solids.

Serve the juice immediately, over ice if desired.

Carrot, Blueberry, and Grape Juice is a nutritious and tasty way to start your day or to refresh yourself after a workout. Carrots provide beta-carotene and other vitamins and minerals, blueberries and grapes add a sweet and fruity flavor to the juice.

Cucumber and Lemon Juice.

Ingredients:

2 medium-sized cucumbers

1 lemon

1 cup of water (optional)

Instructions:

Wash the cucumbers and lemon.

Cut the cucumbers into small pieces that can easily fit into a juicer.

Cut the lemon in half and remove the peel, being careful to remove as much of the white pith as possible.

Put the cucumber pieces into the juicer, followed by the lemon halves.

If desired, add 1 cup of water to the juicer to help the ingredients blend more easily.

Blend the ingredients until they are well combined.

Strain the juice through a fine mesh strainer to remove any solids.

Serve the juice immediately, over ice if desired.

Juicing for Kidney Health

Cucumber and Lemon Juice is a refreshing and healthy way to start your day or to cool down on a hot summer day. Cucumber provides hydration, while the lemon adds a burst of tart flavor.

Lightly Steamed Asparagus and Cucumber Juice.

Ingredients:

1 bunch of asparagus (about 8-10 stalks)

2 medium-sized cucumbers

1 cup of water (optional)

Instructions:

Wash the asparagus and cucumbers.

Cut the tough ends off the asparagus stalks and discard.

Place the asparagus in a steamer basket and lightly steam for about 3-5 minutes, until the asparagus is tender but still crisp.

Let the asparagus cool for a few minutes, then cut into small pieces that can easily fit into a juicer.

Cut the cucumbers into small pieces that can easily fit into a juicer.

Put the asparagus and cucumber pieces into the juicer.

If desired, add 1 cup of water to the juicer to help the ingredients blend more easily.

Blend the ingredients until they are well combined.

Strain the juice through a fine mesh strainer to remove any solids.

Serve the juice immediately, over ice if desired.

The Lightly Steamed Asparagus and Cucumber Juice is a nutritious and refreshing way to start your day or to refresh yourself after a workout. Asparagus provides vitamins and minerals, while

Juicing for Kidney Health

the other fruit provides hydration. The light steaming helps to preserve the delicate flavor of the asparagus, making for a unique and delicious juice.

Apple and Cinnamon Juice.

Ingredients:

4 medium-sized apples (red delicious, granny smith, or a combination of both)

1 cinnamon stick

1 tablespoon of honey (optional)

1 cup of water

Instructions:

Wash the apples and remove the stem and seeds.

Cut the apples into small pieces.

In a saucepan, bring water to a boil. Add the cinnamon stick and let it simmer for 5 minutes.

Add the apple pieces to the cinnamon water and let it boil for 10 minutes, or until the apples are soft.

Remove from heat and let it cool for a few minutes.

Transfer the mixture to a blender and blend until smooth.

Strain the mixture through a fine-mesh strainer to remove any solids and fibers.

If desired, add honey to taste. Stir until well combined.

Pour the apple and cinnamon juice into glasses and serve immediately.

Enjoy your Apple and Cinnamon Juice

Juicing for Kidney Health

Carrot, Ginger, and Turmeric Juice

Ingredients:

4 medium-sized carrots, peeled and chopped

1 inch piece of fresh ginger, peeled and chopped

1 inch piece of fresh turmeric, peeled and chopped

1 lemon, juiced

1 cup of water

Instructions:

Wash the carrots, ginger, and turmeric.

Cut the carrots into small pieces.

In a blender, combine the carrots, ginger, turmeric, lemon juice, and water.

Blend the mixture on high speed for 2-3 minutes, or until smooth.

Strain the mixture through a fine-mesh strainer to remove any solids and fibers.

Pour the Carrot, Ginger, and Turmeric Juice into glasses and serve immediately.

Grapefruit and Mint Juice.

Ingredients:

2 medium-sized grapefruits, peeled and segmented

1/4 cup of fresh mint leaves

1/2 lemon, juiced

1 tablespoon of honey (optional)

1 cup of water

Juicing for Kidney Health

Instructions:

Wash the grapefruits and mint leaves.

Cut the grapefruits into small pieces.

In a blender, combine the grapefruit pieces, mint leaves, lemon juice, honey (if using), and water.

Blend the mixture on high speed for 2-3 minutes, or until smooth.

Strain the mixture through a fine-mesh strainer to remove any solids and fibers.

Pour the Grapefruit and Mint Juice into glasses and serve immediately.

Cucumber and Ginger Juice.

Ingredients:

2 medium-sized cucumbers, peeled and chopped

1 inch piece of fresh ginger, peeled and chopped

1/2 lemon, juiced

1 tablespoon of honey (optional)

1 cup of water

Instructions:

Wash the cucumbers and ginger.

Cut the cucumbers into small pieces.

In a blender, combine the cucumber pieces, ginger, lemon juice, honey (if using), and water.

Blend the mixture on high speed for 2-3 minutes, or until smooth.

Strain the mixture through a fine-mesh strainer to remove any solids and fibers.

Juicing for Kidney Health

Pour the Cucumber and Ginger Juice into glasses and serve immediately.

Enjoy your hydrating and energizing Cucumber and Ginger Juice

Carrot and Lemon Juice.

Ingredients:

4 large carrots, peeled and chopped

1 large lemon, peeled and seeded

2 inches of fresh ginger, peeled

1/2 teaspoon honey (optional)

Pinch of salt

Instructions:

Wash and chop the carrots into small pieces.

Peel and seed the lemon.

Peel the ginger and chop it into small pieces.

Add the chopped carrots, lemon, and ginger to a blender.

Blend the ingredients until they are smooth.

Strain the mixture through a fine mesh strainer to remove any fibers or seeds.

Add a pinch of salt and optional honey to taste.

Stir to combine and serve immediately.

Drink your fresh and healthy Carrot and Lemon Juice

Juicing for Kidney Health

Apple and Parsley Juice.

Ingredients:

4 large apples, cored and chopped

2 cups fresh parsley leaves, washed and dried

1 lemon, peeled and seeded

1 inch of fresh ginger, peeled (optional)

1/2 teaspoon honey (optional)

Pinch of salt

Instructions:

Wash, core, and chop the apples into small pieces.

Wash and dry the parsley leaves.

Peel and seed the lemon.

Peel and chop the ginger into small pieces, if using.

Add the apples, parsley, lemon, and ginger (if using) to a blender.

Blend the ingredients until they are smooth.

Strain the mixture through a fine mesh strainer to remove any fibers or seeds.

Add a pinch of salt and optional honey to taste.

Stir to combine and serve immediately.

Drink your fresh and healthy Juice.

Juicing for Kidney Health

Cucumber and Celery Juice.

Ingredients:

2 medium cucumbers, peeled and chopped

4 large stalks of celery, washed and chopped

1 lemon, peeled and seeded

1 inch of fresh ginger, peeled (optional)

1/2 teaspoon honey (optional)

Pinch of salt

Instructions:

Wash, peel, and chop the cucumbers into small pieces.

Wash and chop the celery into small pieces.

Peel and seed the lemon.

Peel and chop the ginger into small pieces, if using.

Add the cucumbers, celery, lemon, and ginger (if using) to a blender.

Blend the ingredients until they are smooth.

Strain the mixture through a fine mesh strainer to remove any fibers or seeds.

Add a pinch of salt and optional honey to taste.

Stir to combine and serve immediately.

Enjoy your fresh and healthy Cucumber and Celery Juice

Juicing for Kidney Health

Carrot, Pineapple, and Ginger Juice.

Ingredients:

4 large carrots, peeled and chopped

1 cup fresh pineapple, peeled and chopped

1 inch of fresh ginger, peeled

1/2 teaspoon honey (optional)

Pinch of salt

Instructions:

Wash and chop the carrots into small pieces.

Peel and chop the pineapple into small pieces.

Peel and chop the ginger into small pieces.

Add the carrots, pineapple, and ginger to a blender.

Blend the ingredients until they are smooth.

Strain the mixture through a fine mesh strainer to remove any fibers or seeds.

Add a pinch of salt and optional honey to taste.

Stir to combine and serve immediately.

Drink your fresh and healthy Carrot, Pineapple, and Ginger Juice

Lightly Steamed Green Beans and Cucumber Juice.

Ingredients:

1 cup green beans, washed and trimmed

2 medium cucumbers, peeled and chopped

Juicing for Kidney Health

1 lemon, peeled and seeded

1 inch of fresh ginger, peeled (optional)

1/2 teaspoon honey (optional)

Pinch of salt

Instructions:

Wash and trim the green beans.

Lightly steam the green beans for about 5 minutes or until tender but still crisp.

Allow the green beans to cool.

Peel and chop the cucumbers into small pieces.

Peel and seed the lemon.

Peel and chop the ginger into small pieces, if using.

Add the green beans, cucumbers, lemon, and ginger (if using) to a blender.

Blend the ingredients until they are smooth.

Strain the mixture through a fine mesh strainer to remove any fibers or seeds.

Add a pinch of salt and optional honey to taste.

Stir to combine and serve immediately.

Enjoy your Juice

Apple, Beet, and Ginger Juice.

Ingredients:

4 medium apples, cored and chopped

1 medium beet, peeled and chopped

Juicing for Kidney Health

1 inch of fresh ginger, peeled

1/2 lemon, peeled and seeded

1/2 teaspoon honey (optional)

Pinch of salt

Instructions:

Wash, core, and chop the apples into small pieces.

Peel and chop the beet into small pieces.

Peel and chop the ginger into small pieces.

Peel and seed the lemon.

Add the apples, beet, ginger, and lemon to a blender.

Blend the ingredients until they are smooth.

Strain the mixture through a fine mesh strainer to remove any fibers or seeds.

Add a pinch of salt and optional honey to taste.

Stir to combine and serve immediately.

Enjoy your Apple, Beet, and Ginger Juice

Step-by-step instructions for making fresh, homemade juice using a juicer or blender.

Wash and prepare the fruits and vegetables. Thoroughly wash the fruits and vegetables to eliminate any dirt or debris. Peel or slice the ingredients into small pieces that will fit through the feed tube of your juicer or blender.

Assemble the juicer or blender. Assemble the juicer or blender according to the manufacturer's instructions.

Juicing for Kidney Health

In a juicer or blender, combine the following ingredients: Depending on the sort of juicer or blender you have, you may need to feed the ingredients through the feed tube one piece at a time. If using a blender, you may wish to add extra liquid (such as water or juice) to help the ingredients blend more smoothly.

Turn on the juicer or blender, and process the ingredients until they are fully juiced or blended. When using a juicer, the juice will come out of one end and the pulp will come out of the other. If you use a blender, the mixture will be smooth.

Strain the juice (if using a blender): If using a blender, strain the mixture through a fine mesh strainer to remove any fibers or seeds.

Season the juice with salt, honey, or other ingredients to taste. Stir everything together. Serve the juice right away, over ice if desired.

Note: Depending on the type of juicer or blender you have, you may need to employ different procedures to get the best results. It's a good idea to consult the manufacturer's instructions for particular instructions for your equipment.

Safety guidelines for those with kidney disease.

If you have kidney disease, you should be cautious about the ingredients in your juices because certain foods and beverages can be harmful to your kidney health. Here are some safety precautions to take:

Ingredients high in potassium should be avoided: Potassium is a mineral that is required for various bodily activities. However, if you have a kidney illness, your kidneys may be unable to adequately eliminate extra potassium from your body, resulting in excessive potassium levels (hyperkalemia). Potassium-rich foods include bananas, oranges, potatoes, spinach, and tomatoes. To lower your chances of having hyperkalemia, avoid these juice additives.

Limit your sodium intake. Sodium is a mineral that helps your body regulate fluid balance. If you have kidney disease, your kidneys may be unable to adequately remove extra sodium, resulting in high blood pressure and fluid buildup. To help reduce your sodium levels, restrict

Juicing for Kidney Health

your intake of high-sodium meals and beverages, such as processed and packaged foods and juices with added salt.

Select low-protein ingredients: If you have severe renal disease, you may need to limit your protein consumption to make your kidneys work less hard. Cucumbers, carrots, green beans, and apples are examples of low-protein foods.

Consult your doctor: Before making any dietary changes, you should consult with your doctor. Based on your individual health needs and medical history, your doctor may propose a specific diet plan for you.

You may help safeguard your kidney health and enjoy the many advantages of fresh, homemade juices by following these safety tips. Just make sure to consult with your doctor first and make any required changes based on your individual health requirements.

Tips for optimizing the health benefits of juice.

Some guidelines should be followed in order to properly maximize the health benefits of juice.

Use organic ingredients: Organic fruits and vegetables are devoid of potentially dangerous chemicals and pesticides found in non-organic produce. These hazardous elements can impair one's health and diminish the nutritional value of the juice.

Fresh juice should be consumed within 24 hours. Freshly squeezed juice contains the highest concentration of vitamins, minerals, and antioxidants. Juice begins to lose nutritional value as soon as it is created, so drink it within 24 hours of making it.

Consume juice in moderation: While juice might be a healthy alternative, keep in mind that it still includes natural sugars and should be eaten in moderation. Drinking too much juice might result in an excessive sugar intake, which can be hazardous to one's health. Juice should be consumed in moderation as part of a balanced diet, with no more than 1-2 glasses consumed per day.

Use a variety of fruits and vegetables: Using a variety of fruits and vegetables in your juice will provide you with the most comprehensive range of nutrients. Dark leafy greens, brilliantly

Juicing for Kidney Health

colored fruits, and root vegetables are examples of this. This will help to guarantee that your juice is high in vitamins, minerals, and antioxidants.

Consider adding more ingredients: To enhance the health benefits of your juice, consider including ingredients such as ginger, turmeric, or lemon. These additives can enhance the flavor of your juice while also providing health advantages such as lowering inflammation, boosting the immune system, and improving digestion.

In summary, including juice in your diet can be an excellent way to improve your health and well-being. By following these guidelines, you may maximize the health advantages of juice and guarantee that you get the most nutrients from each glass.

Ideas for incorporating juice into a well-balanced diet.

Juicing can be an excellent method to include more fruits and vegetables in your diet, which is beneficial to general health and wellness, including kidney health. Here are some suggestions for including juice in a healthy diet:

Use juice as a supplement to entire fruits and vegetables: While juice can be a terrific method to get a concentrated dosage of nutrients, keep in mind that it lacks the fiber found in full fruits and vegetables. So, instead of replacing complete fruits and veggies in your diet, use juice as a complement.

Choose low-potassium fruits and vegetables: If you have kidney problems, you should limit your potassium intake. Bananas, oranges, avocados, and potatoes are examples of potassium-rich foods and vegetables. Berries, apples, carrots, and celery are all low-potassium foods. You can prepare juice with these low-potassium options and add them to your diet.

Limit added sugar: Limiting added sugar in your diet is crucial since too much sugar can be damaging to your health, especially if you have renal problems. Avoid adding extra sugar to your juice by using naturally sweet fruits like berries or apples.

Consider juicing with greens: dark leafy greens are high in vitamins and minerals while being low in potassium. Greens like spinach, kale, and chard can be added to your juice for a concentrated dosage of these nutrients.

Juicing for Kidney Health

Try mixing and matching different ingredients to make your juice more interesting and to ensure you're getting a variety of nutrients. You may make a juice using apples, carrots, and ginger, or berries, spinach, and lemon, for example.

Juice should be consumed in moderation. While juice might be a healthy alternative, it's vital to remember that it includes natural sugars, and ingesting too much of it can be hazardous to your health. Limit your juice usage to 1-2 glasses per day and consume it as part of a balanced diet.

In essence, including juice in your diet can be an excellent approach to improving your overall health and fitness, including kidney health. You can get the most out of your juice and promote your general well-being by following these suggestions and being careful of your overall diet.

Juicing for Kidney Health

CHAPTER 8

Incorporating Juicing into a Healthy Lifestyle

Juicing as part of a healthy lifestyle can have a significant impact on kidney health. Because the kidneys filter waste products from the body, it is critical to support their function through a healthy diet and lifestyle. It is a simple and delicious way to accomplish this.

It allows you to consume a concentrated amount of nutrients from fruits and vegetables, providing your kidneys with the vitamins, minerals, and antioxidants they require to function optimally. Antioxidants found in many fruits and vegetables, for example, can help protect the kidneys from oxidative stress, which is a major cause of kidney disease.

It also help kidney health by reducing the workload on the kidneys in addition to providing key nutrients. Many juices are low in sodium and high in potassium, two important electrolytes that help the body maintain fluid balance. This can help to relieve strain on the kidneys, which are in charge of removing excess sodium from the body. Juicing can also help to increase fluid intake, which is essential for keeping the kidneys hydrated and functioning properly.

However, it is important to note that not all juices are created equal when it comes to supporting kidney health. Some juices, especially those high in sugar or containing added sugars, can be harmful to the kidneys and increase the risk of kidney disease. Choose fresh, whole foods over juices that are high in sugar, artificial sweeteners, or preservatives.

In conclusion, incorporating juicing into a healthy lifestyle can benefit kidney health. It can help to support overall kidney function and reduce the risk of kidney disease by providing the kidneys with the nutrients they require, reducing the workload on the kidneys, and increasing fluid intake. Making healthy, nutrient-rich juices a part of your daily routine can help to keep your kidneys healthy and improve your overall well-being.

Sarah, is a 42-year-old office worker who has been suffering from kidney disease for several years. Her doctor had diagnosed her with chronic kidney disease and told her that she needed to make some lifestyle changes to slow the progression of the disease.

Juicing for Kidney Health

She had always been interested in natural remedies and alternative forms of healing, so she was intrigued when she learned about the benefits of juicing for kidney health. She decided to give it a shot and started including fresh juices in her diet.

She initially found juicing to be a bit overwhelming. She had no idea what ingredients to use or how to flavor the juices. But she didn't give up and kept trying different combinations of ingredients until she found one she liked. She began with simple ingredients such as carrots, apples, and ginger before gradually incorporating more nutrient-dense fruits and vegetables such as spinach, kale, and beets.

Sarah began to notice significant changes in her health as she continued to juice. Throughout the day, her energy levels increased, and she felt more alert and focused. She also noticed that her digestion had improved, and she was no longer suffering from the bloating and discomfort that she had been experiencing for years.

The most significant improvement was in her kidney health. Sarah's kidney function had been gradually declining for years, but after incorporating juicing into her diet, she was surprised to discover that it had actually improved. She was overjoyed to have discovered a natural way to support her kidney health and slow the progression of her disease.

She continued to juice on a regular basis and discovered that it had become an important part of her healthy lifestyle. She no longer felt overwhelmed and stressed about her health, but rather empowered and in command. She had discovered a simple and delicious way to improve her kidney health and overall well-being.

Finally, Sarah's story demonstrates that incorporating juicing into a healthy lifestyle can have a significant impact on kidney health. It is possible to improve overall kidney function and quality of life by making simple and healthy dietary changes. Anyone, including Sarah, can begin incorporating juicing into their diet and reap the many benefits it has to offer.

Choosing the Right Ingredients

Choosing the right juice ingredients is an important part of incorporating juicing into a healthy lifestyle. The flavor, nutrient content, and overall health benefits of your juice will be determined

Juicing for Kidney Health

by the ingredients you use. To maximize the benefits of juicing, select ingredients that are high in vitamins, minerals, antioxidants, and other nutrients that are necessary for good health.

There are numerous fruits and vegetables that are ideal for juicing, each with its own set of health benefits. Apples, carrots, spinach, kale, beets, ginger, and citrus fruits are all popular ingredients. Experiment with various ingredients to find the combinations that you enjoy the most.

When selecting ingredients for your juice, keep the nutrient content of each in mind. For example, spinach is an excellent juicing ingredient because it is high in vitamins A, C, and K, as well as antioxidants and iron. Kale, on the other hand, is an excellent juicing ingredient due to its high calcium, potassium, and magnesium content. Ginger is also an excellent addition to your juice because it has anti-inflammatory properties and can aid digestion.

In addition to selecting ingredients based on their nutrient content, consider the flavor of each ingredient. Some ingredients, such as beets, have a strong flavor that may not appeal to everyone. It's critical to strike a balance between nutrient-dense ingredients and those you enjoy eating.

To find the right ingredient balance, start with a base of mild-flavored ingredients, such as apples or carrots, and then add in more flavorful ingredients, such as ginger or beets, to taste. This allows you to personalize your juice while still reaping the health benefits of the ingredients you choose.

Finally, choosing the right juice ingredients is an important part of incorporating juicing into a healthy lifestyle. To ensure that you're getting the most out of your juice, consider the nutrient content, flavor, and overall health benefits of each ingredient. You can find the perfect combination for you by experimenting with different ingredients and reaping all of the benefits of juicing.

Making juicing a daily habit.

Making juicing a daily habit is a critical step toward incorporating it into a healthy lifestyle. You can reap the numerous health benefits of juicing by incorporating it into your daily routine.

Juicing for Kidney Health

Making a new habit, on the other hand, can be difficult, so having a plan in place to help you stick to it is essential.

Setting aside a specific time each day for juicing is one of the best ways to make juicing a daily habit. This could be your first thing in the morning, a mid-morning or afternoon snack, or even part of your evening routine. Setting a specific time each day will increase your chances of making juicing a regular part of your routine.

Setting goals for yourself is another way to make juicing a daily habit. Begin by juicing once a day and gradually increasing the frequency as you become more comfortable with the process. This will not only help you stick with your new habit, but it will also allow you to track your progress and see how far you've come.

Another critical aspect of making juicing a daily habit is planning ahead. Make sure you have all of the necessary ingredients on hand, and schedule enough time each day to juice and clean up. It will be easier to stick to your new habit if you have a well-stocked pantry and a plan in place.

Making juicing a social experience is also important. Encourage your friends and family to join you on your juicing journey, or join a local juicing club to meet others who want to incorporate juicing into a healthy lifestyle. Not only will this make juicing more enjoyable, but it will also provide you with a support system to help you stay on track.

In summary, incorporating juicing into a healthy lifestyle requires making it a daily habit. You can make juicing a regular part of your routine and enjoy all of the health benefits it has to offer by setting aside a specific time each day, setting goals, planning ahead, and making it a social experience.

Finding a juicing routine that works for you.

Juicing has grown in popularity as a way for many people to get more nutrients and vitamins into their diets. Fresh, homemade juices can be a tasty and convenient way to support your overall health, including kidney health. With so many different fruits and vegetables to choose from, it can be difficult to know where to begin and how to develop a juicing routine that works best for you.

Juicing for Kidney Health

Before you start juicing, you should understand the function of your kidneys in your body. Your kidneys are vital organs that aid in the removal of waste and excess fluids from your blood. They also help to produce hormones that regulate blood pressure and promote bone health by regulating the levels of various minerals and chemicals in your blood.

It is critical to support your kidney health by eating a healthy diet rich in fruits and vegetables and staying hydrated. Juicing can be an excellent way to accomplish this, as long as you use the proper ingredients.

Some fruits and vegetables are especially beneficial when it comes to juicing for kidney health. Beets, for example, are high in nitrates, which have been shown to help maintain healthy blood pressure and improve blood flow to the kidneys. Cucumbers are also beneficial to kidney health because they are a good source of hydration and can aid in the removal of waste and toxins from the body. Other fruits and vegetables that are good for kidney health are:

Berries: Berries high in antioxidants, such as blueberries, raspberries, and blackberries, can help support healthy kidney function.

Leafy greens, such as kale, spinach, and chard, are high in vitamins and minerals, including potassium, which is essential for kidney function.

Citrus fruits, such as lemons, limes, and oranges, are high in vitamin C and citric acid, which can aid in kidney function.

Carrots are high in vitamins and minerals, including potassium, and can aid in kidney function.

When it comes to incorporating these ingredients into your juicing routine, experiment to see what works best for you. For example, you could start your day with a glass of beet, cucumber, and lemon juice, or you could add berries and leafy greens to your juice throughout the day.

It's also important to remember that, while juicing can be an excellent way to support kidney health, it's only one component of a well-rounded diet. Consume a variety of other fruits and vegetables, whole grains, lean proteins, and healthy fats, as well as plenty of water throughout the day.

In conclusion, developing a juicing routine that works for you can be a tasty and convenient way to support your kidney health. You can help ensure that your kidneys are functioning optimally

Juicing for Kidney Health

by incorporating kidney-friendly fruits and vegetables into your diet, such as beets, cucumbers, leafy greens, citrus fruits, and carrots. Remember to experiment to find out what works best for you and to eat a well-balanced diet and stay hydrated for optimal kidney health.

Incorporating juicing into meals.

Juicing your meals can be a great way to improve your overall health, including your kidney health. Fresh, homemade juices can provide your body with essential vitamins, minerals, and nutrients, which can help improve kidney function and protect your overall health.

Before incorporating juicing into your diet, you should first understand the function of your kidneys in your body. Your kidneys are vital organs that aid in the removal of waste and excess fluids from your blood. They also help to produce hormones that regulate blood pressure and promote bone health by regulating the levels of various minerals and chemicals in your blood.

It is critical to select the right ingredients when juicing to support kidney health. Fruits and vegetables high in vitamins, minerals, and antioxidants are especially good for kidney health. Beets, for example, are high in nitrates, which have been shown to help maintain healthy blood pressure and improve blood flow to the kidneys. Cucumbers are also beneficial to kidney health because they are a good source of hydration and can aid in the removal of waste and toxins from the body.

It is as simple as adding a glass of fresh juice to your breakfast or as a snack throughout the day to incorporate these ingredients into your juicing routine. Juicing can also be incorporated into your meals by using freshly made juices as a base for smoothies or to add flavor and nutrients to soups, sauces, and marinades.

For example, you could start your day with a glass of beet, cucumber, and lemon juice, or you could make a healthy breakfast smoothie with freshly squeezed orange juice. You can also include fresh juices in your meals by using them as the liquid in a soup or sauce or by marinating chicken or fish in them.

When incorporating juicing into your meals, it's important to consider portion sizes and frequency in addition to choosing the right ingredients. Even when made from natural sources,

Juicing for Kidney Health

juices are often high in sugar, so it's important to limit your intake and balance your juicing with a healthy diet that includes plenty of whole foods and hydration.

Incorporating juice into your meals can be an excellent way to support kidney health. You can help ensure that your kidneys are functioning optimally and that you are protecting your overall health by selecting the right ingredients and being mindful of portion sizes and frequency. So why not start juicing with your meals today and see the results for yourself?

Making Juicing a Social Experience.

Making juicing a social experience can enhance its enjoyment. Juicing with friends, family, or community members allows you to not only share the benefits of juicing but also to bond over a common interest.

There are numerous ways to make juicing a social activity. One option is to host a juice party with friends and family. You can all get together, choose ingredients, and take turns making and tasting various juices. This can be a fun way to learn about new recipes and ingredients while also sharing your favorite juicing tips.

Joining a juicing group or club is another way to make juicing a social experience. Local groups can be found through social media, community centers, and health food stores. These organizations frequently organize events like group juice cleanses, tastings, and workshops where you can learn about juicing and meet new people who share your interests.

Participating in a juice fast or cleanse with friends or family members can also make juicing a social experience. This can be a great way to support and hold each other accountable during the process. Furthermore, you can compare notes and share your experiences, which will make the process more enjoyable and manageable.

If you have children, you can include them in your juicing routine. You can teach them about the advantages of juicing, the value of eating fruits and vegetables, and how to make their own juices. This can be a fun and educational experience that encourages your children to form healthy habits that will benefit them for the rest of their lives.

Juicing for Kidney Health

Finally, you can socialize juicing by hosting a juicing-themed event, such as a juice bar at a party, a juice-making competition, or a juicing workshop. This can be a fun way to get people interested in juicing, try new recipes and ingredients, and connect with others who have similar interests.

Finally, making juicing a social experience can enhance its enjoyment and benefits. There are many ways to turn juicing into a social experience that can bring people together and promote health and wellness, whether you organize a juicing party with friends, join a juicing group, participate in a juice fast or cleanse with others, involve your children, or host a juicing-themed event. So, try making juicing a social experience today and reap the benefits.

Tips for Success

Experimenting with Different Ingredients.

Juicing with different ingredients can be a fun and effective way to support kidney health. Juicing allows you to easily consume a variety of high-nutrient fruits, vegetables, and herbs, which can help to support healthy kidney function. The possibilities for delicious and healthy juices are endless with so many ingredients to choose from.

One of the best things about juicing is that you can experiment with different ingredients and flavors without worrying about the texture. If you don't like the taste of kale or spinach, you can add them to your juice along with other ingredients you like, such as apples, carrots, or ginger, to make a delicious and nutritious juice.

Here are some ingredients to try in your juicing routine to improve kidney health:

Cucumber: Cucumbers are an excellent juicing ingredient because they are high in water content and can aid in the removal of toxins from the kidneys. They are also low in potassium, which is important for those who suffer from kidney disease.

Beetroot: High in antioxidants, beetroot can help to improve blood flow and reduce inflammation throughout the body, including the kidneys.

Juicing for Kidney Health

Cranberries are high in antioxidants and can help prevent urinary tract infections, which can strain the kidneys.

Garlic is a potent ingredient that can help improve kidney function by reducing inflammation and increasing blood flow.

Ginger is a natural anti-inflammatory that can help reduce swelling and promote healthy kidney function.

Lemons are high in vitamin C and can aid in the removal of toxins from the kidneys. They also help to alkalinize the body, which can be beneficial for those suffering from kidney disease.

Pomegranate: High in antioxidants, pomegranates can help reduce inflammation and improve blood flow in the kidneys.

Turmeric is a potent anti-inflammatory that can help reduce swelling and improve kidney function.

When experimenting with different ingredients, keep in mind that some fruits and vegetables contain high levels of potassium or phosphorus, which can be harmful to people who have kidney problems. Bananas, avocados, and oranges, for example, are high in potassium, whereas nuts and dairy products are high in phosphorus.

Before beginning a new juicing routine, consult with your healthcare provider, especially if you have any underlying health conditions. Your healthcare provider can advise you on which ingredients are safe to include in your juicing routine and make personalized recommendations based on your specific health needs.

Juicing with different ingredients can be a fun and effective way to support your kidney health. The possibilities are endless with so many ingredients to choose from, and you can find the perfect combination of ingredients to suit your individual tastes and health needs.

Incorporating Whole Foods into Your Diet.

Including whole foods in your diet is an important step toward a healthy and balanced diet. Whole foods are unprocessed or minimally processed foods that contain a high concentration of nutrients, fiber, and other health-promoting compounds. By incorporating more whole foods into your diet, you can reap the many benefits of a whole-foods-rich diet, such as increased energy, better digestion, and a lower risk of chronic diseases.

So, what exactly are whole foods? Fruits, vegetables, whole grains, legumes, nuts, seeds, and lean proteins are examples of whole foods. These foods have been minimally processed and do not contain any added sugars, unhealthy fats, or artificial ingredients. Consuming these foods will provide your body with essential vitamins, minerals, antioxidants, and fiber, which will help you maintain good health.

One advantage of eating whole foods is that they are low in calories while being high in nutrients. This makes them ideal for those trying to maintain or lose weight because they help control appetite and provide sustained energy throughout the day. Whole foods are also high in fiber, which is necessary for good digestion and the prevention of chronic diseases like heart disease and type 2 diabetes.

Another advantage of eating whole foods is that they contain a high concentration of antioxidants and phytochemicals, which help protect the body from oxidative stress and chronic diseases. Consuming a diet high in fruits and vegetables, for example, has been linked to a lower risk of cancer, heart disease, and other chronic illnesses.

It is simple and easy to incorporate whole foods into your diet. Here are some pointers to get you started:

Plan your meals: Spend some time planning your meals and snacks for the week, and make sure to include a variety of whole foods at each meal.

Shop for whole foods: When you go grocery shopping, look for whole foods like fruits, vegetables, whole grains, and lean proteins. Processed and packaged foods should be avoided because they are often high in added sugars, unhealthy fats, and artificial ingredients.

Cook at home: Cooking at home allows you to have complete control over the ingredients in your meals. Try to prepare meals with fresh, whole foods as much as possible, and avoid processed foods as much as possible.

Juicing for Kidney Health

Experiment with new foods: try new whole foods and new recipes that use these ingredients. This can help keep your meals interesting and prevent diet boredom.

Limit your intake of added sugars and unhealthy fats, such as those found in processed and packaged foods, and instead choose healthier fat sources, such as those found in nuts, seeds, and avocados.

Including whole foods in your diet is an important step toward a healthy and balanced diet. With so many advantages, there's no reason not to begin incorporating more whole foods into your diet right away. Begin experimenting with new recipes and ingredients.

Making Gradual Changes.

Making gradual diet changes is an effective way to achieve long-term and sustainable results. Instead of making drastic changes to your diet all at once, making small, gradual changes over time can help you stick to healthier habits and achieve your goals in a realistic and manageable manner.

Here are some suggestions for making gradual diet changes:

Begin Small: Each week or month, make small, manageable dietary changes. Begin by substituting water for sugary drinks or a piece of fruit for a processed snack. As you become more comfortable with healthier habits, you can make additional changes to your diet.

Maintain a Food Journal: Maintaining a food journal can assist you in keeping track of what you eat and identifying areas where you can make changes. Make a list of everything you eat and drink, including portion sizes and when you eat it.

Instead of focusing on what you can't eat, focus on adding more whole foods to your diet, such as fruits, vegetables, whole grains, and lean proteins. You will naturally reduce your intake of unhealthy foods if you focus on adding healthy foods.

Plan Your Meals and Snacks: Plan your meals and snacks ahead of time to ensure you have healthy options on hand when you need them. Keep healthy snacks on hand, such as fruit, nuts, or cut-up vegetables, in case you get hungry in between meals.

Juicing for Kidney Health

Increase Physical Activity Gradually: In addition to making dietary changes, gradually increasing your physical activity can help you achieve your weight loss goals and improve your overall health. Begin with short, daily walks of 10-15 minutes and gradually increase the duration and intensity of your physical activity as you gain fitness.

Be patient: change takes time, so be patient and persistent. Remember that small, gradual changes add up over time and that you are moving in the direction of a healthier, happier life.

Celebrate Your Victories: Celebrate your victories along the way, no matter how small. Recognizing your progress can help you stay motivated and on track toward your objectives.

Making gradual diet changes is a practical and effective way to achieve your health and weight loss objectives. You can make lasting changes to your habits and live a healthier, happier life by taking small, manageable steps toward a healthier diet.

Including whole foods in your diet is an important step toward a healthy and balanced diet. Whole foods are unprocessed or minimally processed foods that contain a high concentration of nutrients, fiber, and other health-promoting compounds. By incorporating more whole foods into your diet, you can reap the many benefits of a whole-foods-rich diet, such as increased energy, better digestion, and a lower risk of chronic diseases.

So, what exactly are whole foods? Fruits, vegetables, whole grains, legumes, nuts, seeds, and lean proteins are examples of whole foods. These foods have been minimally processed and do not contain any added sugars, unhealthy fats, or artificial ingredients. Consuming these foods will provide your body with essential vitamins, minerals, antioxidants, and fiber, which will help you maintain good health.

One advantage of eating whole foods is that they are low in calories while being high in nutrients. This makes them ideal for those trying to maintain or lose weight because they help control appetite and provide sustained energy throughout the day. Whole foods are also high in fiber, which is necessary for good digestion and the prevention of chronic diseases like heart disease and type 2 diabetes.

Another advantage of eating whole foods is that they contain a high concentration of antioxidants and phytochemicals, which help protect the body from oxidative stress and chronic diseases.

Juicing for Kidney Health

Consuming a diet high in fruits and vegetables, for example, has been linked to a lower risk of cancer, heart disease, and other chronic illnesses.

It is simple and easy to incorporate whole foods into your diet. Here are some pointers to get you started:

Plan your meals: Spend some time planning your meals and snacks for the week, and make sure to include a variety of whole foods at each meal.

Shop for whole foods: When you go grocery shopping, look for whole foods like fruits, vegetables, whole grains, and lean proteins. Processed and packaged foods should be avoided because they are often high in added sugars, unhealthy fats, and artificial ingredients.

Cook at home: Cooking at home allows you to have complete control over the ingredients in your meals. Try to prepare meals with fresh, whole foods as much as possible, and avoid processed foods as much as possible.

Experiment with new foods: try new whole foods and new recipes that use these ingredients. This can help keep your meals interesting and prevent diet boredom.

Limit your intake of added sugars and unhealthy fats, such as those found in processed and packaged foods, and instead choose healthier fat sources, such as those found in nuts, seeds, and avocados.

Including whole foods in your diet is an important step toward a healthy and balanced diet. With so many advantages, there's no reason not to begin incorporating more whole foods into your diet right away. Begin experimenting with new recipes and ingredients to reap the many benefits of a whole-foods diet.

Incorporating juicing into a healthy lifestyle can provide a number of advantages, ranging from improved digestion and increased energy levels to an improvement in overall health and wellness. Here's a rundown of the main advantages of juicing:

Increased Nutrient Intake: Juicing is a quick and easy way to up your intake of fruits and vegetables, which are essential components of a healthy diet. You can easily consume the

Juicing for Kidney Health

recommended daily amount of fruits and vegetables by juicing, which can benefit your overall health and wellness.

Improved Digestion: Juicing can aid digestion by providing your body with a concentrated source of nutrients that are easier to absorb. The fiber and pulp from fruits and vegetables are removed, leaving only the liquid, making it easier for your body to absorb and utilize the nutrients.

Enhanced Energy: Juicing can help you feel more energized by providing your body with a quick source of vitamins, minerals, and antioxidants. Fruits and vegetables contain concentrated nutrients that can help boost your overall energy levels, leaving you feeling refreshed and revitalized.

Cleansing and detoxification: Juicing can help cleanse and detoxify your body by providing a concentrated source of nutrients that aid in the removal of toxins and impurities. This can help to improve your overall health and wellness, as well as digestion, energy levels, and skin clarity.

Weight management can be aided by incorporating juicing into a healthy diet and providing your body with a source of low-calorie, nutrient-dense foods. Juicing can help you feel fuller and more satisfied with your meals, which can help you lose weight by reducing your overall calorie intake.

Improved Immune System: Juicing can help boost your immune system by providing your body with a concentrated source of vitamins, minerals, and antioxidants. These nutrients can help boost your immune system, allowing you to fight off illness and disease.

Juicing is a quick, convenient, and accessible way to increase your intake of fruits and vegetables, even if you have a hectic schedule. Juicing takes only a few minutes, and the resulting juice can be taken with you on the go, making it a convenient option for those who are always on the go.

Incorporating juicing into a healthy lifestyle can provide a number of advantages, ranging from improved digestion and increased energy levels to an improvement in overall health and wellness. It can be a convenient and effective way to achieve your goals, whether you want to improve your health, lose weight, or simply consume more fruits and vegetables.

Juicing for Kidney Health

A Delectable and Fun Way to Improve Your Health: Juicing is a delectable and enjoyable way to improve your overall health and wellness. With so many fruits, vegetables, and herbs to choose from, you can play around with different ingredients and flavors until you find the perfect combination for you.

Juicing is a great way to improve your overall health and wellness. Juicing can be a convenient and effective way to achieve your goals, whether you want to increase your energy levels, improve your digestion, or simply consume more fruits and vegetables. So, why bother? Begin juicing today and reap the numerous benefits.

Finally, consider the gradual changes that can be made when incorporating juicing into a healthy lifestyle. Making gradual changes can help to ensure a manageable and sustainable transition. Whether you are just starting out or have been juicing for a while, going slowly and making small changes over time can help you stick with your juicing routine and reap the many benefits that it offers.

Incorporating juicing into a healthy lifestyle can be an extremely effective way to improve your overall health and wellness. There is no better time to start juicing than now, with all of the benefits it offers, including increased intake of fruits and vegetables, cleansing and detoxification, convenience and accessibility, and a fun and delicious way to improve your health. So, consider the advantages of juicing, make gradual changes, and begin juicing today.

Juicing for Kidney Health

The kidneys are one of the most vital organs in our bodies. These bean-shaped organs in the lower back are in charge of filtering waste products and excess fluids from the blood. They also play an important role in electrolyte regulation, blood pressure control, and the production of hormones that regulate red blood cell production and promote strong bones. Optimal kidney health is critical for overall health and well-being. Unfortunately, many people take their kidneys for granted and fail to give them the attention they require until they begin to fail.

However, by following a few simple guidelines, you can keep your kidneys healthy and functioning properly.

Overview of the importance of kidney health.

It is impossible to overestimate the significance of kidney health. Our kidneys play an important role in our overall health and well-being. These vital organs filter waste and excess fluids from the blood, regulate electrolyte levels, control blood pressure, and produce hormones that regulate red blood cell production and promote strong bones.

The body cannot function properly without healthy kidneys. Waste products and excess fluids can accumulate in the blood, causing a variety of health issues. Furthermore, because the kidneys play an important role in blood pressure regulation, damage to these organs can result in high blood pressure and an increased risk of heart disease and stroke.

Kidney disease is a serious and growing public health issue. Over 30 million people in the United States have chronic kidney disease, and millions more are at risk. Unfortunately, kidney disease is frequently misdiagnosed until it has progressed to a serious stage, so it's critical to be aware of the risk factors and take precautions to protect your kidney health.

Diabetes, high blood pressure, a family history of kidney disease, and being over 60 are all risk factors for kidney disease. If you have any of these risk factors, you should have your kidneys

Juicing for Kidney Health

checked by a healthcare provider on a regular basis. Early detection and treatment of kidney disease can help slow its progression and avoid serious health complications.

The role of the kidneys in maintaining overall health.

The kidneys play an important role in our overall health and well-being. These vital organs are found in the lower back and are in charge of a variety of important functions that keep our bodies running smoothly.

The kidneys' primary function is to filter waste products and excess fluids from the blood. The kidneys filter the blood constantly, removing waste products and excess fluids and excreting them from the body in the form of urine. This contributes to keeping the blood clean and free of harmful substances, which is critical for overall health and well-being.

In addition to filtering waste and excess fluids, the kidneys play an important role in electrolyte regulation. Electrolytes are minerals that are essential for many bodily functions, such as muscle and nerve function, hydration, and blood pressure regulation. The kidneys assist in electrolyte regulation by filtering them from the blood and excreting any excess.

The kidneys also play an important role in blood pressure regulation. The kidneys produce hormones that help regulate blood pressure and aid in the removal of excess salt from the body. This helps to maintain healthy blood pressure, lowering the risk of heart disease and stroke.

It produces hormones that regulate red blood cell production and promote bone strength. Erythropoietin, one of these hormones, stimulates the production of red blood cells, which transport oxygen to the body's tissues. Calcitriol is another hormone that helps regulate calcium levels in the body and promotes strong bones.

The kidneys are important for maintaining the body's fluid balance. They assist in maintaining the proper fluid balance by retaining water when the body is dehydrated and excreting water when there is an excess. This keeps the body hydrated and running smoothly.

Finally, they play an important role in overall health and well-being. These vital organs filter waste and excess fluids, regulate electrolyte levels, control blood pressure, produce hormones that regulate red blood cell production and promote strong bones, and regulate fluid balance in

Juicing for Kidney Health

the body. Maintaining optimal kidney health and taking care of your kidneys is critical for overall health and well-being.

The impact of diet on kidney health.

Diet is essential for maintaining kidney health because the foods we eat can either help or harm our kidneys, it's critical to make informed food choices. In this article, we'll look at how diet affects kidney health and what you can do to maintain optimal kidney function.

Blood pressure is one of the primary ways that diet influences kidney health. Hypertension, or high blood pressure, is a major risk factor for kidney disease. A high-salt, processed-food diet can raise blood pressure and place undue strain on the kidneys. A low-salt diet rich in fresh fruits, vegetables, and whole grains, on the other hand, can help maintain healthy blood pressure levels and reduce the risk of kidney disease.

The amount of protein in your diet is another important factor to consider when it comes to diet and kidney health. Protein is necessary for good health, but too much of it can be harmful to the kidneys. It's especially important to limit your protein intake if you have chronic kidney disease because your kidneys can't filter excess protein as well. Your healthcare provider can assist you in determining the appropriate amount of protein for your specific needs.

Aside from salt and protein, diet can have an impact on kidney health by influencing blood sugar levels. Diabetics are more likely to develop kidney disease, and a diet high in sugar and processed foods can make it difficult to control blood sugar levels. A diet high in whole grains, fruits, and vegetables, on the other hand, can help keep blood sugar levels in check and reduce the risk of kidney disease.

Staying hydrated is critical for good kidney health. Water consumption can help flush waste products and excess fluids from the kidneys, lowering the risk of kidney disease. Aim for at least 8 glasses of water per day, and more if you are active or live in a hot climate.

Finally, diet is critical to maintaining optimal kidney health. A low-salt diet rich in whole grains, fruits, and vegetables, as well as adequate protein and hydration, can help protect your kidneys and lower your risk of kidney disease. Talk to your healthcare provider if you have any concerns

Juicing for Kidney Health

about your kidney health. They can assist you in developing a healthy eating plan that is tailored to your specific requirements.

Role of exercise in maintaining kidney health.

Exercise is an important part of overall health and wellness, and it is no different when it comes to kidney health. Our kidneys are responsible for filtering waste and excess fluids from our bloodstream, regulating blood pressure, and balancing electrolyte levels in our bodies. It is critical to maintain them in order to avoid potential damage and ensure that they function properly. Exercise can help with this goal in a variety of ways.

To begin with, regular exercise can help you maintain a healthy weight, which is essential for kidney health. Obesity is a major risk factor for chronic kidney disease (CKD), and it can cause kidney damage over time. Excess calories are burned and fat stores are reduced when you exercise. As a result, the strain on the kidneys is reduced, and the risk of CKD is reduced.

It also help to regulate blood pressure, which is another important factor in kidney health. High blood pressure, also known as hypertension, is a major cause of CKD and can damage the delicate blood vessels in the kidneys over time. Regular exercise can help lower blood pressure by increasing circulation and decreasing stress, both of which are factors that contribute to hypertension.

Aside from these advantages, exercise can help improve heart health, which is closely related to kidney health. The heart and kidneys collaborate to regulate blood flow and keep the cardiovascular system running smoothly. Exercise can improve heart health by strengthening the heart muscle and increasing circulation into kidney health. The heart and kidneys collaborate to regulate blood flow and keep the cardiovascular system running smoothly. Exercise can improve heart health by strengthening the heart muscle and increasing circulation. This, in turn, can aid in kidney protection and reduce the risk of damage.

Furthermore, exercise can help regulate the levels of various electrolytes in the body, which is important for kidney health. Electrolytes such as sodium, potassium, and calcium are essential

Juicing for Kidney Health

for the proper functioning of the body's various systems, including the kidneys. Regular exercise can help regulate these levels by promoting electrolyte and fluid balance in the body.

Finally, it helps to reduce stress, which is important for overall health, including kidney health. Stress can cause the body to produce hormones and chemicals that are harmful to the kidneys and other organs. Exercise can help reduce stress by releasing endorphins and improving mood, both of which can benefit kidney health.

Finally, exercise is an important part of maintaining kidney health. Exercise can help prevent kidney damage and ensure optimal kidney function by regulating weight, blood pressure, heart health, electrolyte levels, and stress. To support kidney health and promote overall well-being, it is critical to incorporate regular physical activity into your routine.

Recommendations for physical activity and its impact on kidney function.

Physical activity is critical to overall health and wellness, and it is no different when it comes to kidney health. Regular exercise can improve kidney function by preventing damage and ensuring optimal performance. In this article, we'll go over some of the most important physical activity recommendations and how they affect kidney function.

First and foremost, moderate-intensity physical activity for at least 30 minutes five days a week is advised. This can include brisk walking, cycling, swimming, or any other type of aerobic exercise. This level of physical activity can help you maintain a healthy weight, control your blood pressure, and improve your heart health, all of which are important for your kidneys.

Strength training, such as weightlifting or resistance band exercises, should be added to your routine in addition to aerobic exercise. Strength training can aid in the development and maintenance of muscle mass, which is essential for maintaining a healthy weight and lowering the risk of chronic kidney disease (CKD).

It is also critical to be mindful of the type and intensity of physical activity, especially for those suffering from kidney disease. High-impact activities, such as running or jumping, can be difficult on the kidneys and can result in additional strain or damage. Before beginning a new

Juicing for Kidney Health

exercise routine, consult with your healthcare provider, especially if you have a history of kidney disease or other health conditions.

Furthermore, hydration is an important aspect of physical activity and has an impact on kidney function. Hydration is essential for the kidneys to function properly, so drink plenty of fluids before, during, and after exercise. It's also a good idea to avoid dehydrating drinks like alcohol and sugary drinks, which can be bad for your kidneys.

Exercise can also help reduce stress, which is important for overall health, including kidney health. Stress can cause the body to produce hormones and chemicals that are harmful to the kidneys and other organs. Exercise can help reduce stress by releasing endorphins and improving mood, both of which can benefit kidney health.

In summary, physical activity is critical to maintaining kidney health. Individuals can help prevent kidney damage and ensure optimal kidney function by engaging in moderate-intensity physical activity for at least 30 minutes five days a week, incorporating strength training, being mindful of the type and intensity of physical activity, staying hydrated, and reducing stress. To support kidney health and promote overall well-being, it is critical to incorporate regular physical activity into your routine.

The benefits of regular physical activity for overall health.

Physical activity is an important part of living a healthy lifestyle. It provides numerous advantages that improve our overall health, both physically and mentally. In this sub-chapter, we will look at the various ways that regular physical activity benefits our health.

Improves Cardiovascular Health: Improving cardiovascular health is one of the most significant advantages of regular physical activity. Exercise strengthens the heart and blood vessels, lowering the risk of heart disease, stroke, and high blood pressure. Physical activity also improves blood circulation, lowering the risk of blood clots and other related problems.

Strengthens Bones and Muscles: Regular physical activity aids in the development and maintenance of strong bones and muscles. This is especially important as we get older because

Juicing for Kidney Health

our bones and muscles naturally weaken. Running, jumping, and weightlifting are all weight-bearing exercises that help stimulate bone growth and prevent osteoporosis.

Weight Control: Regular physical activity is an effective way to maintain a healthy weight. Exercise increases muscle mass and burns calories, which can boost the metabolism and aid in weight loss. Regular physical activity can also help reduce the risk of obesity and other health problems.

Improves Mental Health: Regular physical activity is beneficial not only to the body but also to the mind. Exercise has been shown to alleviate stress, anxiety, and depression while also improving mood and cognitive function. It also encourages better sleep, which is critical for overall mental health.

Improves Immunity: Regular physical activity strengthens the immune system, lowering the risk of illness and infection. Exercise increases blood flow, allowing the body to deliver essential nutrients and oxygen to cells, including immune cells. This can aid in reducing inflammation and improving the body's ability to fight infections.

Regular physical activity has been shown to improve digestive health by encouraging regular bowel movements and lowering the risk of constipation. Exercise also lowers the risk of colorectal cancer by decreasing inflammation and oxidative stress in the body.

Increases Energy Levels: Physical activity on a regular basis can boost energy levels, making it easier to get through the day. Exercise increases the production of endorphins, which are natural pain relievers and mood boosters that leave you feeling energized and alert.

Finally, regular physical activity is an important part of living a healthy lifestyle. It has numerous advantages, including better cardiovascular health, stronger bones and muscles, weight management, mental health, improved immunity, digestive health, and increased energy levels. For the best health outcomes, incorporate physical activity into your daily routine, whether it's through a structured workout or simply going for a walk.

Juicing for Kidney Health

The impact of chronic health conditions on kidney health.

Chronic health problems can have a big impact on kidney health and function. The kidneys are responsible for filtering waste products from the blood as well as regulating fluid levels, electrolyte balance, and blood pressure. Chronic health conditions can harm the kidneys and cause them to fail over time. Let's look at how some of the most common chronic health conditions affect kidney health.

Diabetes is a chronic disease that impairs the body's ability to regulate blood sugar levels. High blood sugar levels can damage the blood vessels in the kidneys over time, reducing their ability to filter waste from the blood. This can result in kidney disease, also known as diabetic nephropathy, which is one of the leading causes of kidney failure.

High blood pressure, also known as hypertension, is a common chronic health condition that affects the kidneys' health. High blood pressure places additional strain on the blood vessels in the kidneys, reducing their ability to filter waste from the blood. This can cause kidney damage and an increased risk of kidney failure over time.

Heart Disease: Conditions such as coronary artery disease and heart attacks can have an impact on kidney health. The heart and kidneys collaborate to keep the body's fluid levels, electrolyte balance, and blood pressure in check. When the heart isn't working properly, it can interfere with the kidneys' ability to filter waste products from the blood.

Chronic kidney disease (CKD) is a condition in which the kidneys gradually lose function over time. Diabetes, high blood pressure, and heart disease are all risk factors for chronic kidney disease. When the kidneys aren't working properly, they can't filter waste from the blood, which increases the risk of kidney failure.

Polycystic kidney disease is a genetic condition in which cysts form in the kidneys, reducing their ability to filter waste products from the blood. Cysts can enlarge over time, causing kidney damage and increasing the risk of kidney failure.

Lupus is an autoimmune disease that can affect a variety of organs, including the kidneys. Lupus can cause kidney inflammation, reducing their ability to filter waste products from the blood. Lupus can cause kidney failure in severe cases.

Juicing for Kidney Health

Chronic Liver Disease: Conditions such as hepatitis and cirrhosis, as well as chronic liver disease, can have an impact on kidney health. The liver and kidneys collaborate to keep the body's fluid levels, electrolyte balance, and blood pressure in check. When the liver isn't working properly, it can interfere with the kidneys' ability to filter waste products from the blood.

Finally, chronic illnesses can have a significant impact on kidney health and function. Diabetes, high blood pressure, heart disease, chronic kidney disease, polycystic kidney disease, lupus, and chronic liver disease are just a few of the many chronic health conditions that can harm the kidneys and impair their ability to filter waste products from the blood. If you have a chronic health condition, it is critical that you work with your doctor to manage your condition and protect your kidney health. This may include changes in your lifestyle, medication, and regular monitoring of your kidney function.

The importance of managing chronic health conditions.

Chronic health problems, such as high blood pressure and diabetes, are becoming more common in our society. These conditions can have a significant impact on overall health and well-being, and if not properly managed, they can lead to serious health problems. The importance of managing chronic health conditions and how to do so effectively are as follows:

The Importance of Blood Pressure Management: Hypertension, also known as high blood pressure, is a common chronic health condition that affects millions of people worldwide. High blood pressure, if left untreated, can lead to serious health problems such as heart disease, stroke, and kidney damage. High blood pressure can be effectively managed with lifestyle changes such as a healthy diet, regular physical activity, stress management, and medication.

Diabetes Management: Diabetes is a chronic disease that impairs the body's ability to regulate blood sugar levels. Diabetes, if left untreated, can cause serious health problems such as heart disease, nerve damage, and kidney damage. Diabetes can be effectively managed through a combination of lifestyle changes, such as a healthy diet and regular physical activity, and medication.

Juicing for Kidney Health

Changes in Lifestyle for Better Health: Lifestyle changes such as a healthy diet and regular physical activity can help manage chronic health conditions. A nutritious diet high in fruits, vegetables, whole grains, and lean proteins can help regulate blood sugar levels and lower blood pressure. Walking, cycling, or swimming on a regular basis can help reduce stress and improve overall health.

Importance of Medication: Medication can also play an important role in managing chronic health conditions. In the case of high blood pressure and diabetes, for example, medication can be prescribed to lower blood pressure and regulate blood sugar levels. Working with your healthcare provider to determine the best medication regimen for your specific needs and regularly monitoring your health to ensure that your condition is properly managed is critical.

Regular monitoring and check-ups with your healthcare provider can help you manage chronic health conditions. Your healthcare provider can assess your condition, monitor any changes, and make any necessary adjustments to your treatment plan during these check-ups. Regular monitoring can also aid in the early detection of potential health issues, allowing for prompt and effective treatment.

Finally, managing chronic health conditions such as high blood pressure and diabetes is critical for overall health and well-being. A healthy diet and regular physical activity, as well as medication, can help with effective management. Regular monitoring and check-ups with your healthcare provider can also help to ensure that your condition is well-managed and that any potential health problems are identified early. You can protect your health and live a longer, healthier life by taking a proactive approach to managing your chronic health conditions.

Role of medication and lifestyle changes.

Medication and lifestyle changes are critical in the management of chronic health conditions like high blood pressure, diabetes, and heart disease. If left untreated, these conditions can lead to serious health problems and a lower quality of life. Here, we will look at the role of medication and lifestyle changes in managing chronic health conditions, as well as how they can be combined effectively for optimal health.

Juicing for Kidney Health

Medication is frequently prescribed to help manage chronic health conditions like high blood pressure and diabetes. Blood pressure medications, such as ACE inhibitors and diuretics, for example, can be used to lower blood pressure and reduce the risk of heart disease and stroke. Diabetes medications, such as metformin and sulfonylureas, can also be used to control blood sugar levels and prevent complications from developing.

Changes in Lifestyle such as a healthy diet and regular physical activity can also play an important role in the management of chronic health conditions. A nutritious diet high in fruits, vegetables, whole grains, and lean proteins can help regulate blood sugar levels and lower blood pressure. Walking, cycling, or swimming on a regular basis can help reduce stress and improve overall health.

Individuals with chronic health conditions can benefit from a healthy lifestyle in a variety of ways. A healthy diet, for example, can help to regulate blood sugar levels and lower blood pressure, lowering the risk of heart disease and stroke. Physical activity on a regular basis can also help to reduce stress, improve overall health, and improve quality of life.

Combining medication with lifestyle changes is important. Combining medication and lifestyle changes can be an effective way to manage chronic health conditions. Medication can be used to treat the underlying condition, while lifestyle changes like a healthy diet and regular physical activity can help to improve overall health and lower the risk of complications.

Routine monitoring and check-ups with your healthcare provider can be extremely beneficial for managing chronic health conditions. Your healthcare provider can assess your condition, monitor any changes, and make any necessary adjustments to your treatment plan during these check-ups. Regular monitoring can also aid in the early detection of potential health issues, allowing for prompt and effective treatment.

Finally, both medication and lifestyle changes are important in managing chronic health conditions such as high blood pressure and diabetes. A healthy lifestyle, which includes a nutritious diet and regular physical activity, can improve overall health and lower the risk of complications. Combining medication and lifestyle changes can help manage chronic health conditions and improve quality of life.

Juicing for Kidney Health

Regular monitoring and check-ups with your healthcare provider can also help to ensure that your condition is well-managed and that any potential health problems are identified early. You can protect your health and live a longer, healthier life by taking a proactive approach to managing your chronic health conditions.

Importance of regularly monitoring kidney function.

Kidneys are vital organs that play an important role in overall health. They are in charge of removing waste and excess fluids from the body, balancing electrolytes, and producing hormones that control blood pressure and promote red blood cell production. Kidney function must be monitored on a regular basis due to its critical role in health maintenance. This section will provide an overview of the importance of regularly monitoring kidney function and the methods for doing so.

Early Detection of Kidney Disease: Regular monitoring of kidney function can aid in the early detection of any potential issues, allowing for prompt and effective treatment. Early detection of kidney disease can help to prevent or delay disease progression, lowering the risk of serious health problems and improving quality of life.

Monitoring Treatment Effectiveness: Regular monitoring of kidney function can also aid in determining the effectiveness of kidney disease treatment. Monitoring kidney function allows healthcare providers to assess treatment response, make necessary adjustments, and monitor any changes in the condition.

Regular monitoring of kidney function can assist in assessing kidney function over time, allowing healthcare providers to detect any changes or trends in the condition. This information can be used to make future treatment decisions and to determine the best course of action for maintaining kidney health.

Complications: Regular monitoring of kidney function can also aid in the detection of potential complications such as anemia, high blood pressure, and bone disease, all of which are common in people with kidney disease. When these complications are detected early, healthcare providers can provide prompt and effective treatment, lowering the risk of serious health problems.

Juicing for Kidney Health

Assessing the Need for Dialysis or a Kidney Transplant: In individuals with advanced kidney disease, regular monitoring of kidney function can also help to assess the need for dialysis or a kidney transplant. Monitoring kidney function allows healthcare providers to determine when dialysis or a kidney transplant is required, as well as provide appropriate treatment to keep the kidneys healthy.

Methods of Monitoring Kidney Function: Blood and urine tests, imaging tests, and kidney function tests are all available for monitoring kidney function. Creatinine, a waste product of muscle metabolism, and urea, a waste product of the liver, are both indicators of kidney function and can be measured using blood and urine tests. Ultrasound, CT scan, and MRI imaging tests can be used to visualize and assess the kidneys' structure and function. Kidney function tests, such as the glomerular filtration rate (GFR) test, can be used to determine how much waste and fluid the kidneys filter.

Finally, regular monitoring of kidney function is critical for maintaining kidney health and avoiding serious health issues. Regular monitoring can assist in detecting potential problems early, assessing treatment effectiveness, monitoring kidney function over time, detecting potential complications, and determining the need for dialysis or a kidney transplant. Healthcare providers can provide appropriate treatment and support to maintain kidney health and improve quality of life by monitoring kidney function.

Common tests used to monitor kidney function.

Monitoring kidney function is an important part of overall health maintenance and preventing serious health problems. Blood tests, urine tests, imaging tests, and kidney function tests are some of the tests that can be used to monitor kidney function. In this article, we will discuss some of the most common tests used to monitor kidney function.

Blood tests are used to measure creatinine and urea levels, which are waste products produced by the body. Creatinine and urea levels in the blood can indicate a decline in kidney function. The creatinine clearance test is a common blood test that measures how much creatinine the kidneys remove from the blood. This test determines the kidneys' ability to filter waste and excess fluids from the body.

Juicing for Kidney Health

Urine tests are used to determine the amount and concentration of waste products in the urine. These tests can help determine whether or not the kidneys are working properly and identify any potential problems, such as an increased risk of kidney disease, urinary tract infections, and other conditions that may affect kidney function. Urine tests can also be used to evaluate the efficacy of kidney disease treatment.

Imaging tests, such as ultrasound, CT scans, and MRIs, can be used to visualize and assess the kidneys' structure and function. These tests can aid in the detection of potential issues such as cysts, tumors, and other conditions that may impair kidney function. Imaging tests can also be used to track the progression of kidney disease and evaluate treatment efficacy.

Kidney Function Tests: Kidney function tests, such as the glomerular filtration rate (GFR), can be used to determine how much waste and fluid the kidneys filter. The GFR test is the most accurate way to determine kidney function because it measures the kidneys' ability to filter waste and excess fluids from the blood. A low GFR indicates a decline in kidney function, whereas a high GFR indicates normal kidney function.

A biopsy is a test in which a small sample of kidney tissue is removed for examination under a microscope. This test can be used to diagnose kidney disease and determine its severity. The results of a biopsy can also be used to decide on the best course of treatment for kidney disease.

Blood tests, urine tests, imaging tests, kidney function tests, and biopsies are some of the tests that can be used to monitor kidney function. These tests can provide valuable information about kidney function and aid in the early detection of potential problems, allowing for prompt and effective treatment. Individuals can maintain kidney health and reduce the risk of serious health problems by regularly monitoring kidney function.

The role of regular check-ups and health screenings.

Regular check-ups and health screenings are critical for maintaining kidney health and avoiding serious health issues. Individuals who regularly monitor their health can identify potential problems early on and take the necessary steps to address them. This chapter will go over the significance of regular check-ups and health screenings in maintaining kidney health.

Juicing for Kidney Health

Kidney Disease Early Detection: Kidney disease is a common condition that frequently goes undetected until it has progressed to an advanced stage. Regular check-ups and health screenings can aid in the early detection of kidney disease, when it is easier to treat and manage. Blood and urine tests can be used to evaluate kidney function and identify any potential issues, such as an increased risk of kidney disease, urinary tract infections, and other conditions that may impair kidney function.

Chronic health conditions such as high blood pressure and diabetes are common risk factors for kidney disease and should be monitored. Regular check-ups and health screenings can aid in tracking the progression of these conditions and determining the efficacy of treatment. Blood and imaging tests can be used to evaluate kidney function and detect any potential problems associated with chronic health conditions.

Assessing Treatment Effectiveness: Regular check-ups and health screenings can aid in determining the effectiveness of treatment for kidney disease and other conditions that may impair kidney function. Blood tests, urine tests, and imaging tests can all be used to track the progression of kidney disease and evaluate treatment effectiveness. This data can be used to make any necessary treatment changes and ensure that individuals receive the best possible care.

Maintaining a Healthy Lifestyle: Regular check-ups and health screenings can also assist people in maintaining a healthy lifestyle and lowering their risk of serious health problems. Individuals who regularly monitor their health can identify potential problems early on and take the necessary steps to address them. Making dietary changes, increasing physical activity, quitting smoking, and managing stress are all examples of this.

Monitoring for Complications: Regular check-ups and health screenings can also aid in the detection of potential complications associated with kidney disease and other conditions that may impair kidney function. Individuals with kidney disease, for example, may be more likely to develop heart disease, anemia, and other serious health issues. Regular check-ups and health screenings can assist in detecting these complications early on and addressing them.

Regular check-ups and health screenings are critical for maintaining kidney health and avoiding serious health issues. Individuals who regularly monitor their health can identify potential problems early on and take the necessary steps to address them. Regular check-ups and health

Juicing for Kidney Health

screenings can also aid in assessing treatment effectiveness, maintaining a healthy lifestyle, and monitoring for potential complications. Individuals can ensure that they receive the best possible care and maintain their kidney health over time by prioritizing regular check-ups and health screenings.

Avoiding Harmful Substances.

The impact of harmful substances on kidney health.

By filtering waste and excess fluids from the bloodstream, the human kidneys play an important role in overall health. However, a variety of harmful substances, including drugs, chemicals, and other toxic substances, can harm the kidneys. In this article, we will look at the effects of harmful substances on kidney health and the importance of avoiding these substances whenever possible.

Nonsteroidal anti-inflammatory drugs (NSAIDs) such as ibuprofen, as well as certain antibiotics, can be harmful to the kidneys. These drugs can harm the kidneys by decreasing blood flow to them, reducing their ability to filter waste and excess fluids from the bloodstream. Furthermore, some medications, such as angiotensin-converting enzyme inhibitors (ACE inhibitors), can harm the kidneys by altering blood flow to the kidneys.

Chemicals: Chemicals such as lead, mercury, and solvents can be toxic to the kidneys. These chemicals can harm the kidneys by interfering with their ability to filter waste and excess fluids from the bloodstream, resulting in a buildup of harmful substances in the bloodstream. Furthermore, chemical exposure can increase the risk of developing kidney cancer and other serious health problems.

Excessive alcohol consumption can harm the kidneys and raise the risk of kidney disease. Alcohol can harm the kidneys by decreasing blood flow to them, reducing their ability to filter waste and excess fluids from the bloodstream. Furthermore, alcohol can increase the risk of developing serious health problems such as liver disease and pancreatitis, both of which can impair kidney function further.

Smoking is also harmful to the kidneys and raises the risk of kidney disease. Smoking can harm the kidneys by decreasing blood flow to them, reducing their ability to filter waste and excess

Juicing for Kidney Health

fluids from the bloodstream. Furthermore, smoking increases the risk of serious health problems such as cardiovascular disease, which can further impair kidney function.

High levels of salt, animal protein, and processed foods can also be harmful to the kidneys and increase the risk of kidney disease. These dietary factors can harm the kidneys by increasing their workload and impairing their ability to filter waste and excess fluids from the bloodstream.

In summary, the effects of hazardous substances on kidney health can be significant and long-lasting. Drugs, chemicals, alcohol, smoking, and certain dietary factors can all cause kidney damage and impair the kidneys' ability to filter waste and excess fluids from the bloodstream. To support kidney function, it is important to avoid harmful substances whenever possible and to make lifestyle changes, such as eating a healthy diet and engaging in regular physical activity. Regular check-ups and health screenings can also aid in monitoring kidney health and detecting potential problems early on, allowing people to take the necessary steps to address them.

Recommendations for avoiding harmful substances.

Maintaining kidney health is critical for overall health and well-being, and avoiding harmful substances like alcohol and certain medications can help support kidney function. This section will go over recommendations for avoiding harmful substances as well as steps people can take to protect their kidney health.

Excessive alcohol consumption can be harmful to the kidneys and increase the risk of kidney disease. To protect kidney health, it is recommended that women limit their alcohol consumption to one drink per day and men limit their alcohol consumption to two drinks per day. If you have kidney disease, you should avoid alcohol completely.

Caution Should Be Exercised When Using Medications: Certain medications can be harmful to the kidneys and increase the risk of kidney disease. If you take medications on a regular basis, you should talk to your doctor about the potential risks and benefits. Your doctor may be able to suggest alternative medications that are less likely to harm your kidneys.

Avoid using over-the-counter pain relievers: Nonsteroidal anti-inflammatory drugs (NSAIDs) such as ibuprofen, which are available over-the-counter, can be harmful to the kidneys and

Juicing for Kidney Health

increase the risk of kidney disease. If you are in pain, it is critical that you consult with your healthcare provider about alternative treatments.

Avoid Harmful Chemicals: Harmful chemicals such as lead, mercury, and solvents can be harmful to the kidneys and increase the risk of kidney disease. To protect kidney health, avoid exposure to these chemicals as much as possible. If you work in an industry where exposure to hazardous chemicals is unavoidable, it is critical that you follow all safety guidelines and take precautions to protect yourself.

Maintaining a Healthy Diet: A high-salt, animal-protein, and processed-food diet can also be harmful to the kidneys and increase the risk of kidney disease. It is critical to consume a healthy diet rich in fruits, vegetables, whole grains, and lean protein to protect kidney health. Furthermore, it is critical to limit salt, animal protein, and processed foods.

It is critical to avoid harmful substances such as alcohol and certain medications in order to maintain kidney health. Individuals can support kidney function and protect their health for years to come by following these recommendations and making lifestyle changes such as eating a healthy diet and engaging in regular physical activity. Regular check-ups and health screenings can also aid in monitoring kidney health and detecting potential problems early on, allowing people to take the necessary steps to address them.

Dangers of long-term exposure to harmful substances and its effects.

Long-term exposure to hazardous substances can have serious consequences for kidney health, resulting in kidney disease and other related conditions. Here, we will look at the risks of long-term exposure to hazardous substances and how it can affect kidney function.

Harmful Chemicals: Long-term kidney damage can result from exposure to harmful chemicals such as lead, mercury, and solvents. These chemicals can harm the kidney's delicate tissues and cells, resulting in a decline in kidney function over time. Long-term exposure to hazardous chemicals can even cause kidney failure in severe cases.

Prescription Medications: When taken for an extended period of time, certain prescription medications can be harmful to the kidneys. Medication used to treat conditions such as high

Juicing for Kidney Health

blood pressure, heart disease, and pain falls into this category. It is critical to discuss the potential risks and benefits of any medications you are taking with your healthcare provider, as well as to regularly monitor your kidney function.

Over-the-Counter Pain Medications: When taken for an extended period of time, over-the-counter pain medications, such as nonsteroidal anti-inflammatory drugs (NSAIDs), can be harmful to the kidneys. These medications can harm the kidneys' delicate tissues and cells, resulting in a decline in kidney function over time.

Excessive alcohol consumption can be harmful to the kidneys in the long run. Alcohol can harm the delicate tissues and cells in the kidneys, causing kidney function to deteriorate over time. Long-term alcohol consumption can even lead to kidney failure in severe cases.

Poor diet: a diet high in salt, animal protein, and processed foods can also have long-term negative effects on the kidneys. This diet may increase your chances of developing high blood pressure and other conditions that can lead to kidney disease.

It is critical to be aware of the substances to which you are exposed and to take precautions to protect your kidney health. Regular check-ups and health screenings can aid in the early detection of potential problems, allowing people to take the necessary steps to address them. Furthermore, a healthy diet and regular physical activity can help to support kidney function and lower the risk of developing kidney disease. If you have any concerns about your kidney health, you should consult your doctor for a thorough evaluation and treatment plan.

Summary of the tips for maintaining optimal kidney health.

Kidneys are essential for overall health because they filter waste and excess fluids from the blood and regulate electrolyte levels. It is critical to take care of your kidneys in order to prevent or postpone the onset of kidney disease, which can lead to serious health issues. Here is a list of suggestions for maintaining good kidney health.

Drink plenty of water. Water is essential for kidney health. Staying hydrated allows the kidneys to more effectively flush out waste and toxins, lowering the risk of kidney stones and infection.

Juicing for Kidney Health

Regular physical activity can help reduce the risk of developing kidney disease-causing conditions such as high blood pressure, obesity, and diabetes. Aim for 30 minutes of moderate exercise per day, such as brisk walking or cycling.

Maintain good kidney health by eating a healthy diet rich in fruits, vegetables, whole grains, and lean protein. Limit your intake of animal protein and avoid processed and high-sodium foods.

Keep your blood pressure under control: Hypertension is a major risk factor for kidney disease. If you have high blood pressure, it is critical to control it by eating a healthy diet, exercising regularly, and taking medications as directed.

Manage other chronic health conditions: diabetes and heart disease, for example, can increase the risk of developing kidney disease. It is critical to manage these conditions and to have your kidney function checked on a regular basis.

Avoid harmful substances: Excessive alcohol consumption, as well as long-term use of certain medications and pain relievers, can harm the kidneys. It is critical to limit your alcohol consumption and consult with your doctor about the potential risks and benefits of any medications you are taking.

Regular check-ups and health screenings can help detect potential kidney function problems early on, allowing you to take the necessary steps to address them.

You can help to maintain optimal kidney health and lower your risk of developing kidney disease by following these tips and taking care of your kidneys. If you have any concerns about your kidney health, you should consult your doctor for a thorough evaluation and treatment plan.

Final thoughts on the importance of taking care of your kidneys.

The kidneys are vital organs that filter waste and excess fluids from the blood, regulate electrolyte levels, and produce hormones that regulate blood pressure and promote red blood cell production, all of which contribute to overall health. Despite their importance, many people take their kidney health for granted, increasing their risk of kidney disease.

Juicing for Kidney Health

Kidney disease is a serious health issue that can result in a variety of complications, such as anemia, nerve damage, heart disease, and even death. It is a progressive disease, which means that it usually worsens over time and, if left untreated, can lead to kidney failure.

Fortunately, many steps can be taken to prevent or delay the onset of kidney disease, such as:

Maintaining a healthy lifestyle entails eating a balanced diet, exercising regularly, avoiding harmful substances, and managing chronic health conditions such as high blood pressure and diabetes.

Regular kidney function monitoring: Regular check-ups and health screenings can help detect potential kidney function problems early on, allowing you to take the necessary steps to address them.

Speaking with your healthcare provider: If you have any concerns about your kidney health, it is critical that you consult with your healthcare provider for a thorough evaluation and treatment plan.

Taking care of your kidneys is an important part of staying healthy and lowering your risk of developing kidney disease. You can help to ensure optimal kidney health and reduce your risk of developing this serious and potentially life-threatening condition by leading a healthy lifestyle, regularly monitoring your kidney function, and speaking with your healthcare provider.

Encouragement to make positive lifestyle changes.

Maintaining good kidney health is critical for overall health and a high quality of life. The kidneys filter waste and excess fluids from the body, regulate blood pressure, and produce hormones that regulate red blood cell production and promote bone health. However, many factors, such as genetics, unhealthy lifestyle choices, and certain medical conditions, can put stress on the kidneys and cause damage or disease.

Adopting a positive lifestyle that promotes kidney function and reduces the risk of damage is essential for maintaining optimal kidney health. Here are some lifestyle changes you can make to maintain optimal kidney health:

Juicing for Kidney Health

Hydrate on a regular basis: It is critical to drink enough water to keep the kidneys functioning properly. Adequate hydration aids in the removal of waste and toxins from the body, lowering the risk of kidney damage. Aim for 8–10 glasses of water per day, and more if you are physically active.

Eat a balanced and healthy diet: A healthy diet is essential for maintaining optimal kidney health. Reduce your consumption of processed foods, salt, and red meat in favor of fresh fruits and vegetables, whole grains, and lean protein.

Maintain a healthy weight: Being overweight or obese puts additional strain on the kidneys, which can lead to damage and disease. A healthy weight achieved through a balanced diet and regular exercise can help prevent kidney damage and promote optimal kidney health.

Quit smoking and drink less alcohol. Smoking and excessive alcohol consumption are two major risk factors for kidney damage. Quitting smoking and limiting alcohol consumption can reduce the risk of kidney damage and improve kidney function significantly.

Exercise on a regular basis: Maintaining optimal kidney health requires regular exercise. Physical activity helps to regulate blood pressure, relieve kidney stress, and promote overall health. Aim for at least 30 minutes of moderate exercise per week, such as brisk walking.

Control medical conditions: Certain medical conditions, such as diabetes and high blood pressure, can place extra strain on the kidneys, increasing the risk of kidney damage. Controlling these conditions with medication, lifestyle changes, and regular monitoring in collaboration with your healthcare provider can help prevent kidney damage and maintain optimal kidney health.

Regular check-ups with your healthcare provider can help monitor your kidney health and identify any potential problems early. This can aid in the prevention or postponement of kidney damage and promote optimal kidney health.

In summary, positive lifestyle changes to maintain optimal kidney health are critical to overall wellness and a high quality of life. You can reduce the risk of kidney damage and promote optimal kidney function by eating a healthy diet, exercising regularly, and controlling medical

Juicing for Kidney Health

conditions. So, take charge of your kidney health today and make the changes necessary to live a long and healthy life.

Juicing for Kidney Health

CHAPTER 10

Managing Chronic Kidney Disease through Juicing.

Introduction.

Chronic Kidney Disease (CKD) is a progressive condition that affects the kidneys' ability to function. CKD can eventually lead to kidney failure, necessitating dialysis or a kidney transplant. While there is no cure for CKD, proper nutrition and lifestyle changes can assist in managing the condition and slowing its progression. Incorporating juice into your diet is one such change. Juicing is a convenient and tasty way to consume a variety of nutrients, hydrate the body, and support kidney health.

Proper nutrition is essential for people with CKD in order to manage the condition. A healthy diet can help control blood sugar levels, regulate blood pressure, and reduce inflammation and oxidative stress, all of which are important factors in maintaining kidney health. Juicing can be a good way to increase your intake of fruits and vegetables, which are high in vitamins, minerals, and antioxidants that help your kidneys. Juicing can also improve digestion and nutrient absorption, making it easier for the body to utilize the nutrients required to support kidney function.

When juicing with CKD, however, certain precautions must be taken. Certain fruits and vegetables contain high levels of potassium and phosphorus, which can be harmful to people who have kidney disease. To determine the best juices for your specific needs and to ensure you are getting the proper balance of nutrients to support kidney health, consult with a healthcare provider.

You can support kidney health and manage CKD symptoms by incorporating juicing into your diet. Juicing can be an effective way to support your overall health and well-being, whether you want to increase your nutrient intake, hydrate your body, or reduce inflammation. So, start juicing today, and you'll be taking an important step toward managing your CKD.

Juicing for Kidney Health

Chronic Kidney Disease (CKD).

Chronic kidney disease (CKD) is a long-term condition that impairs kidney function. The kidneys are two bean-shaped organs in the lower back that filter waste and excess fluids from the blood, produce urine, and maintain electrolyte balance. They also help to produce hormones that regulate blood pressure, red blood cell production, and calcium metabolism.

It is a progressive disease in which the kidneys are damaged and their ability to function properly deteriorates over time. A variety of factors, including high blood pressure, diabetes, infections, genetics, and certain medications, can cause the damage. When the kidneys are damaged, they are unable to filter waste and excess fluids from the blood, resulting in a toxic build-up in the body.

The severity of CKD varies from mild to severe, and its progression varies from person to person. CKD may not cause any symptoms in its early stages and can go unnoticed for many years. People with the condition may experience fatigue, nausea, loss of appetite, muscle cramps, and swelling in the legs, ankles, and feet as it progresses. CKD can progress to end-stage kidney disease, also known as kidney failure, which necessitates dialysis or a kidney transplant to maintain life.

Early detection and treatment of CKD are critical for slowing its progression and lowering the risk of complications. This includes keeping blood pressure, blood sugar levels, and cholesterol under control, eating a balanced diet, and staying physically active. People with CKD may also need to take medication to control their condition and support kidney function in some cases.

It is a progressive disease that impairs the kidneys' ability to function properly. It is a serious condition that, if not treated properly, can lead to end-stage kidney disease and a variety of other health issues. Early detection and management of CKD, such as a balanced diet and regular medical care, can help slow the progression of the disease and improve quality of life.

Juicing for Kidney Health

Chronic kidney disease (CKD) can have serious consequences for the body and overall health. The kidneys are responsible for filtering waste and excess fluids from the blood, producing urine, and maintaining electrolyte balance. When the kidneys are damaged and their ability to function properly is impaired, waste and fluid buildup in the body can cause a variety of health problems.

One of the most serious consequences of CKD is the accumulation of toxic substances in the body. When the kidneys are damaged, they are unable to filter waste and excess fluids from the blood, resulting in toxic substances such as urea, creatinine, and potassium build-up. This waste build-up can cause fatigue, nausea, and confusion, as well as increase the risk of heart disease, stroke, and other health problems.

CKD can also have serious consequences for the cardiovascular system. The accumulation of waste and fluid in the body can raise blood pressure, increasing the risk of heart disease and stroke. Furthermore, people with CKD are more likely to develop anemia, a condition in which the body does not produce enough red blood cells. This can result in fatigue, weakness, and a decreased ability to engage in physical activity.

CKD can also have an impact on the bones and metabolism. The kidneys play a role in calcium metabolism, and when they are damaged, they may be unable to effectively regulate calcium levels. This can result in osteodystrophy, a condition in which bones become thin, brittle, and fragile. Furthermore, CKD can impair the body's ability to metabolize vitamins and minerals, leading to deficiencies and other health issues.

Finally, CKD can have serious consequences for the nervous system. The accumulation of waste and fluid in the body can damage nerves, causing symptoms such as numbness and tingling in the hands and feet. In severe cases, CKD can also cause pericarditis, which causes inflammation of the heart and causes chest pain and shortness of breath.

In essence, CKD has a significant impact on the body and overall health. Waste and fluid build-up in the body can cause a variety of health issues, including an increased risk of heart disease and stroke, bone problems, and nerve damage. Proper CKD management, which includes a balanced diet and regular medical care, can help reduce the condition's impact on the body and improve quality of life.

Juicing for Kidney Health

Importance of proper nutrition in managing CKD.

Proper nutrition is critical for managing and slowing the progression of chronic kidney disease (CKD). The kidneys are responsible for filtering waste and excess fluids from the blood, producing urine, and maintaining electrolyte balance. A balanced diet that meets the individual's nutritional needs can help support kidney function and overall health when the kidneys are damaged and their ability to function properly is reduced.

A healthy diet for people with CKD should focus on reducing waste and fluid build-up in the body. This may include limiting protein, salt, and potassium intake. People with CKD may also need to limit their intake of phosphorus, a mineral that can build up in the body and cause bone and heart damage.

Aside from limiting certain nutrients, people with CKD must consume adequate amounts of essential nutrients such as iron, calcium, and vitamin D. These nutrients are essential for bone health and overall health. People with CKD may also need to take supplements to ensure they get enough of these nutrients.

Fluid management is also essential in the treatment of CKD. People with CKD may need to limit their fluid intake to avoid fluid build-up and reduce the burden on their kidneys. Fluid-rich foods such as fruits, soups, and stews may be restricted.

Proper nutrition is essential for CKD management and overall health. A well-balanced diet that meets the individual's nutritional needs while limiting waste and fluid build-up in the body is essential. People with CKD should work with a registered dietitian to create a meal plan that meets their nutritional needs while also aiding in the management of their condition. People with CKD can improve their quality of life and slow the progression of their condition with the right dietary approach.

Juicing for Kidney Health

1. Beet Carrot Juice

2. Beet Cucumber Juice

3. Broccoli Carrot Juice

4. Carrot Beet Juice

5. Carrot Celery Juice

6. Carrot Cucumber Juice

7. Carrot Spinach Juice

8. Cabbage Celery Juice

9. Celery Beet Juice

10. Celery Carrot Juice

11. Zucchini Carrot Juice

Apple Juice: Blend 3 medium apples, peeled and cored, with 1 cup of water. Strain through a fine mesh sieve to remove the pulp.

Berry Juice: Blend 1 cup of mixed berries (strawberries, blueberries, blackberries, etc.), 1/2 a banana, and 1/2 cup of water. Strain through a fine mesh sieve to remove the pulp.

Juicing for Kidney Health

Orange Juice: Blend 3 medium oranges, peeled, with 1 cup of water. Strain through a fine mesh sieve to remove the pulp.

Grapefruit Juice: Blend 2 medium grapefruits, peeled and seeded, with 1 cup of water. Strain through a fine mesh sieve to remove the pulp.

Pineapple Juice: Blend 1 medium pineapple, peeled, cored and chopped, with 1 cup of water. Strain through a fine mesh sieve to remove the pulp.

Mango Juice: Blend 1 medium mango, peeled and pitted, with 1 cup of water. Strain through a fine mesh sieve to remove the pulp.

Kiwi Juice: Blend 4 medium kiwis, peeled, with 1 cup of water. Strain through a fine mesh sieve to remove the pulp.

Melon Juice: Blend 1 medium cantaloupe or honeydew melon, peeled and seeded, with 1 cup of water. Strain through a fine mesh sieve to remove the pulp.

Pomegranate Juice: Blend 1 medium pomegranate, seeded, with 1 cup of water. Strain through a fine mesh sieve to remove the pulp.

Lime Juice: Blend 2 medium limes, peeled, with 1 cup of water. Strain through a fine mesh sieve to remove the pulp.

Lemon Juice: Blend 2 medium lemons, peeled, with 1 cup of water. Strain through a fine mesh sieve to remove the pulp.

Peach Juice: Blend 3 medium peaches, pitted and peeled, with 1 cup of water. Strain through a fine mesh sieve to remove the pulp.

Apricot Juice: Blend 3 medium apricots, pitted and peeled, with 1 cup of water. Strain through a fine mesh sieve to remove the pulp.

Juicing for Kidney Health

Cherry Juice: Blend 1 cup of cherries, pitted, with 1/2 cup of water. Strain through a fine mesh sieve to remove the pulp.

Grape Juice: Blend 2 cups of grapes, seeded, with 1/2 cup of water. Strain through a fine mesh sieve to remove the pulp.

Cranberry Juice: Blend 1 cup of cranberries, with 1/2 cup of water. Strain through a fine mesh sieve to remove the pulp.

Strawberry Juice: Blend 1 cup of strawberries, with 1/2 cup of water. Strain through a fine mesh sieve to remove the pulp.

Raspberry Juice: Blend 1 cup of raspberries, with 1/2 cup of water. Strain through a fine mesh sieve to remove the pulp.

Blueberry Juice: Blend 1 cup of blueberries, with 1/2 cup of water. Strain through a fine mesh sieve to remove the pulp.

Blackberry Juice: Blend 1 cup of blackberries, with 1/2 cup of water. Strain through a fine mesh sieve to remove the pulp.

Herb and spice juices (e.g. ginger, turmeric).

Ginger Juice: Blend 1-inch piece of fresh ginger, peeled, with 1 cup of water. Strain through a fine mesh sieve to remove the pulp.

Turmeric Juice: Blend 1-inch piece of fresh turmeric, peeled, with 1 cup of water. Strain through a fine mesh sieve to remove the pulp.

Mint Juice: Blend 1 cup of fresh mint leaves, with 1/2 cup of water. Strain through a fine mesh sieve to remove the pulp.

Juicing for Kidney Health

Basil Juice: Blend 1 cup of fresh basil leaves, with 1/2 cup of water. Strain through a fine mesh sieve to remove the pulp.

Cilantro Juice: Blend 1 cup of fresh cilantro leaves, with 1/2 cup of water. Strain through a fine mesh sieve to remove the pulp.

Parsley Juice: Blend 1 cup of fresh parsley leaves, with 1/2 cup of water. Strain through a fine mesh sieve to remove the pulp.

Dill Juice: Blend 1 cup of fresh dill leaves, with 1/2 cup of water. Strain through a fine mesh sieve to remove the pulp.

Rosemary Juice: Blend 1 cup of fresh rosemary leaves, with 1/2 cup of water. Strain through a fine mesh sieve to remove the pulp.

Sage Juice: Blend 1 cup of fresh sage leaves, with 1/2 cup of water. Strain through a fine mesh sieve to remove the pulp.

Thyme Juice: Blend 1 cup of fresh thyme leaves, with 1/2 cup of water. Strain through a fine mesh sieve to remove the pulp.

Oregano Juice: Blend 1 cup of fresh oregano leaves, with 1/2 cup of water. Strain through a fine mesh sieve to remove the pulp.

Marjoram Juice: Blend 1 cup of fresh marjoram leaves, with 1/2 cup of water. Strain through a fine mesh sieve to remove the pulp.

Bay Leaf Juice: Blend 1 cup of fresh bay leaves, with 1/2 cup of water. Strain through a fine mesh sieve to remove the pulp.

Fennel Juice: Blend 1 cup of fresh fennel fronds, with 1/2 cup of water. Strain through a fine mesh sieve to remove the pulp.

Juicing for Kidney Health

Coriander Juice: Blend 1 cup of fresh coriander leaves, with 1/2 cup of water. Strain through a fine mesh sieve to remove the pulp.

Clove Juice: Blend 1 tsp of whole cloves, with 1/2 cup of water. Strain through a fine mesh sieve to remove the pulp.

Cinnamon Juice: Blend 1 tsp of cinnamon, with 1/2 cup of water. Strain through a fine mesh sieve to remove the pulp.

Nutmeg Juice: Blend 1 tsp of nutmeg, with 1/2 cup of water. Strain through a fine mesh sieve to remove the pulp.

Cardamom Juice: Blend 1 tsp of cardamom, with 1/2 cup of water. Strain through a fine mesh sieve to remove the pulp.

Star Anise Juice: Blend 1 tsp of star anise, with 1/2 cup of water. Strain through a fine mesh sieve to remove the pulp.

Precautions for Juicing with CKD.

Limit fruit juices due to high sugar content.

Fruit juices are frequently seen as a healthy alternative due to the presence of vitamins, minerals, and antioxidants. However, because of the high sugar content, many people with chronic kidney disease (CKD) must limit their intake of fruit juices.

Sugar, commonly known as glucose or fructose, is a carbohydrate that gives the body energy. Sugar, on the other hand, can be harmful to the body in large amounts, particularly for people with CKD. Excess sugar consumption raises the risk of elevated blood sugar levels, which is a major issue for people with renal disease. When the kidneys are not working properly, they are unable to filter out excess sugar, resulting in a buildup of glucose in the blood.

Juicing for Kidney Health

Aside from being heavy in sugar, many fruit juices are also high in calories, which can contribute to weight gain. People with CKD are frequently recommended to maintain a healthy weight in order to lessen the strain on the kidneys and avoid future issues.

Fruit juices include sugar, which can disrupt the mineral balance in the body, which is crucial for people with CKD. High sugar levels, for example, can cause phosphorus buildup in the blood, which can be dangerous for patients with kidney disease. Phosphorus is a mineral that is necessary for healthy bones, but too much of it can create problems such as blood vessel calcification, which can lead to heart disease.

Despite these reservations, fruit juices can be part of a healthy diet for people with CKD. It is vital, however, to limit their use and choose low-sugar alternatives, such as unsweetened 100% fruit juice or diluting regular fruit juice with water. Fresh or unsweetened frozen fruits are also preferred over fruit drinks since they contain the same nutrients with less sugar and are often a better option for those with CKD.

While fruit juices can supply crucial nutrients, patients with CKD should limit their consumption due to the high sugar content. People with CKD can still enjoy the health benefits of fruit while lowering the risk of issues associated with high sugar intake by choosing low-sugar options and fresh or unsweetened frozen fruits.

Avoid juices high in potassium and phosphorus.

People with chronic kidney disease (CKD) should be cautious about the juices they consume since some juices are high in potassium and phosphorus, which can be damaging to their health.

Potassium and phosphorus are important elements for overall health, but in excess, they can be hazardous to people with CKD. The kidneys filter extra potassium and phosphorus from the body, but when they are not working properly, these minerals can build up in the blood and cause issues.

High potassium levels are especially worrisome for people with CKD since they can cause irregular heartbeats and heart failure. People with CKD should limit or avoid drinking juices high in potassium, such as orange, tomato, and prune juice.

Juicing for Kidney Health

High amounts of phosphorus in the blood can lead to a buildup of calcium in the blood vessels, which can contribute to heart disease in people with CKD. Coca-cola, chocolate, and coffee drinks are high in phosphorus and should be reduced or avoided by patients with CKD.

Aside from avoiding potassium and phosphorus-rich liquids, people with CKD can choose low-potassium and low-phosphorus juices like cranberry, grape, and apple juice. However, even these low-potassium and low-phosphorus juices should be drunk in moderation, since they can still contribute to an increase in these minerals if consumed in high quantities.

People with CKD should avoid juices high in potassium and phosphorus and instead pick low-potassium and low-phosphorus choices. They can help to maintain a healthy mineral balance in their bodies and lower the risk of issues connected with excessive levels of potassium and phosphorus by doing so. A healthcare expert should test potassium and phosphorus levels on a regular basis to ensure that they remain within a healthy range.

Check with a healthcare provider before making significant changes to your diet.

Chronic kidney disease (CKD) is a serious ailment that affects millions of individuals around the world and necessitates careful management, including dietary adjustments. While making dietary adjustments can help control symptoms and delay the progression of the disease, it is vital to consult with a healthcare physician before making major changes.

A healthcare specialist, such as a nephrologist or a qualified dietitian, can provide specific advice on appropriate dietary adjustments for you. They can also help you understand which nutrients are vital for your health and which meals to avoid. They can, for example, advise you on the amount of protein, potassium, phosphorus, and other nutrients you should consume on a daily basis as well as how to obtain these elements from your food.

They can help you manage other medical concerns, such as diabetes or high blood pressure, in addition to advising you on the proper nutrients and foods to take. They can also monitor your kidney function and make any necessary adjustments to your medication or treatment plan.

Juicing for Kidney Health

It is also crucial to remember that various people respond differently to dietary changes, and what works for one person may not work for another. Some people, for example, may need to reduce their protein consumption, while others may need to increase it. A healthcare provider can assist you in determining the proper nutrient balance for your specific needs and in making the required dietary changes.

Before making significant dietary changes, consult with your healthcare professional. They can provide specific advice on appropriate dietary modifications for you, check your kidney function, and assist you in managing any other medical disorders that may be present. Working together with a healthcare physician can help you make the proper dietary modifications to manage your CKD and improve your overall health.

Juicing Recipes for People with CKD

Anti-Inflammatory Juice.

If you have Chronic Kidney Disease (CKD), you should eat a diet that promotes kidney health and helps you manage your symptoms. Here are **20 CKD-friendly anti-inflammatory juice recipes** that can help reduce inflammation in the body:

Carrot, Apple, and Ginger Juice

Cucumber, Celery, and Lemon Juice

Blueberry, Blackberry, and Raspberry Juice

Sweet Potato, Carrot, and Ginger Juice

Pineapple, Cucumber, and Lime Juice

Beet, Carrot, and Apple Juice

Spinach, Apple, and Lemon Juice

Juicing for Kidney Health

Avocado, Cucumber, and Lime Juice

Papaya, Mango, and Pineapple Juice

Cabbage, Carrot, and Apple Juice

Cherry, Pomegranate, and Acai Berry Juice

Carrot, Orange, and Ginger Juice

Cucumber, Celery, and Parsley Juice

Broccoli, Cauliflower, and Apple Juice

Kale, Spinach, and Green Apple Juice

Celery, Cucumber, and Lemon Juice

Red Bell Pepper, Tomato, and Carrot Juice

Green Apple, Kiwi, and Spinach Juice

Carrot, Beet, and Ginger Juice

Acai Berry, Blueberry, and Blackberry Juice

It's crucial to remember that some of these substances are high in potassium or phosphorus, which might be dangerous for people with CKD. Before introducing these drinks into your diet, consult with a healthcare physician or a certified dietitian, as they may provide specific advice on what is appropriate for you. You should also reduce your fruit consumption and focus on low-potassium and low-phosphorus items.

Enjoy these anti-inflammatory drinks as part of a balanced and nutritious diet tailored to your specific needs, and always consult with a healthcare provider before making significant dietary changes.

Juicing for Kidney Health

Summary of the benefits of juicing for people with CKD.

Juicing has a lot of advantages for patients with chronic kidney disease (CKD). Here's a rundown of the main advantages of juicing for those with CKD:

1. Increased Nutrient Intake: Juicing can help you consume more vitamins, minerals, and antioxidants, which can benefit your overall health.

2. Improved Hydration: Juices are an excellent source of hydration and can help you stay hydrated and refreshed, especially on hot days.

3. Reduced Inflammation: Anti-inflammatory drinks such as ginger, turmeric, and leafy greens can help reduce inflammation in the body.

4. Better Digestion: By providing the body with easily digestible minerals and fiber, juicing can improve digestion.

5. Increased Energy: Juicing can deliver a rapid energy boost, especially when made with carrots, beets, and apples.

6. Improved Mood: Because of the vitamins, minerals, and antioxidants present in fresh fruits and vegetables, juicing can be a natural and healthy way to boost your mood.

7. Better Sleep: Certain elements in juice, such as chamomile and passion fruit, are believed to help relax the mind and body.

It's crucial to remember that juicing might have side effects for people with CKD, such as being rich in sugar and potassium. Before introducing juicing into your diet, consult with a healthcare physician or a qualified dietitian, as they may provide specific advice on what is best for you. Additionally, focus on low-potassium and low-phosphorus components and restrict your fruit consumption.

Enjoy juicing as part of a balanced and healthy diet tailored to your specific needs, and always consult with a healthcare expert before making substantial dietary changes.

Juicing for Kidney Health

Importance of following a balanced diet and working with a healthcare provider.

Maintaining a healthy diet and working with a healthcare provider are important for anyone, but they are especially important for people with chronic kidney disease (CKD). Here are some of the reasons why people with CKD should eat a balanced diet and cooperate with their healthcare provider:

1.Symptom Management: CKD can cause a number of symptoms such as fatigue, itching, and muscle cramping. A well-balanced diet suited to the needs of people with CKD can help manage these symptoms while also improving general health and well-being.

2. Slowing Condition Advancement: People with CKD can slow the progression of their disease and potentially minimize their risk of complications by eating a balanced diet and engaging with a healthcare provider.

3. Maintaining Optimal Nutrient Levels: People with CKD may need to limit specific nutrients in their diet, such as phosphorus and potassium. A well-balanced diet tailored to their unique needs will help ensure they get the correct balance of nutrients to maintain maximum health.

4. Aiding Treatment: In some circumstances, a balanced diet and collaboration with a healthcare provider can aid in the treatment of CKD. A low-protein diet, for example, may help reduce the course of renal disease.

5.Improving Overall Health: Eating a well-balanced diet and working with a healthcare practitioner can improve overall health by supplying the body with the nutrients and vitamins it requires to function properly.

It is critical to remember that what works for one individual may not work for another. Everyone's needs are unique, and a healthcare physician or qualified dietitian can provide individualized advice on what is best for you. Furthermore, rather than making huge adjustments all at once, it is necessary to make steady and progressive changes to your diet and assess your progress.

Juicing for Kidney Health

In conclusion, patients with CKD should follow a balanced diet and cooperate with a healthcare practitioner to manage symptoms, reduce disease progression, maintain appropriate nutrient levels, aid in therapy, and improve general health. You may improve your health and well-being by making moderate and informed changes to your diet.

Juicing for Kidney Health

CHAPTER 11

Introduction

While there is no cure for CKD at the moment, there are several things that can be done to support kidney health, such as exercise and hydration. In this chapter, we'll discuss the importance of exercise and hydration in maintaining renal health, as well as why they're especially important for people with CKD.

Exercise is an important component of general health and well-being, and it can also improve kidney health. Exercise on a regular basis can improve cardiovascular health, reduce stress and anxiety, increase muscle strength and flexibility, and promote better circulation. Furthermore, exercise can help you maintain a healthy weight, which is vital for kidney health.

Hydration is also an important part of renal health because it aids in kidney function and general health. Staying hydrated can aid in the prevention of dehydration, the prevention of kidney stones, and the promotion of good blood flow. However, it is critical to be aware of the types of beverages consumed, as some can be high in sugar, caffeine, or alcohol, all of which can be harmful to kidney health.

Incorporating exercise and hydration into a complete strategy for CKD management can benefit renal health as well as overall physical and mental well-being. This chapter will look at the benefits of exercise, the forms of exercise that are good for people with CKD, the necessity of hydration, and the fluid consumption that is suggested for CKD patients. Before making significant changes to your exercise or hydration habits, always consult with a healthcare expert, as they may provide specialized advice that is suited for your specific circumstances.

Juicing for Kidney Health

Improved cardiovascular health.

Cardiovascular health is a vital facet of overall health, especially for patients who have chronic kidney disease (CKD). Exercise on a regular basis can help to enhance cardiovascular health, which in turn can help to promote renal health.

Exercise can benefit cardiovascular health in a variety of ways. It can, for example, assist to lower blood pressure, which is a major risk factor for heart disease and stroke. High blood pressure can place additional strain on the heart and blood vessels, as well as contribute to kidney disease. Exercise can assist to reduce the risk of heart disease and stroke by lowering blood pressure, and it can also help to promote kidney function.

Exercise can also help to enhance circulation. Improved circulation can aid in the delivery of oxygen and nutrients to the body's cells, particularly kidney cells. Good circulation can benefit kidney health by allowing them to operate optimally and remove waste products more efficiently.

By strengthening the heart muscle, exercise can also aid to enhance heart health. When you exercise, your heart has to work harder to deliver oxygen and nutrients to your muscles. This can assist to strengthen the heart muscle over time, making it more efficient and lowering the risk of heart disease.

Regular exercise can also help lower cholesterol, which is a major risk factor for heart disease. High cholesterol levels in the blood can contribute to plaque buildup in the arteries, limiting blood flow and increasing the risk of heart disease and stroke. Exercise can help reduce the risk of heart disease and maintain kidney function by lowering cholesterol levels.

It is critical to remember that exercise should be done in moderation and under the supervision of a healthcare expert. Some types of exercise, such as strenuous physical activity or contact sports, may not be suitable for those with CKD. Your healthcare provider may provide you personalized advise on the type and frequency of exercise that is best for you, taking into account your personal health status as well as any other medical concerns you may have.

Juicing for Kidney Health

Finally, good cardiovascular health is a critical component in supporting renal health. Regular exercise can enhance cardiovascular health by lowering blood pressure, increasing circulation, strengthening the heart muscle, and decreasing cholesterol levels. Before making significant changes to your exercise habits, always consult with your healthcare professional to ensure that the fitness program you choose is safe and appropriate for your unique health state.

Better circulation.

Circulation is critical for general bodily health, including the kidneys. Good circulation aids in the delivery of oxygen and nutrients to the body's cells, particularly those in the kidneys, as well as the effective removal of waste products. Improved circulation can help promote kidney health by making them more efficient and lowering the risk of renal disease.

Exercise can aid with circulation in a variety of ways. When you exercise, for example, your heart has to work harder to pump blood to your muscles. This enhanced cardiac output may aid in the improvement of circulation throughout the body, especially to the kidneys. Furthermore, when you exercise, your muscles contract and relax, which helps increase blood flow and lower the risk of blood clots.

Increased circulation can also aid in the reduction of inflammation throughout the body. Many chronic diseases, including kidney disease, are exacerbated by inflammation. Improved circulation can help lower the risk of renal disease and maintain kidney function by reducing inflammation.

Exercise on a regular basis can also help lower blood pressure, which is another condition that can lead to impaired circulation. High blood pressure can make blood flow across the body more challenging, including to the kidneys. Exercise can help to enhance circulation and kidney function by lowering blood pressure.

It is critical to remember that exercise should be done in moderation and under the supervision of a healthcare expert. Some types of exercise, such as strenuous physical activity or contact sports, may not be suitable for those with chronic kidney disease (CKD). Your healthcare provider may provide you with personalized advice on the type and frequency of exercise that is best for you,

Juicing for Kidney Health

taking into account your personal health status as well as any other medical concerns you may have.

Finally, improved circulation is a crucial part of maintaining kidney function. Regular exercise can help improve circulation by boosting cardiac output, decreasing inflammation, and lowering blood pressure.

Reduced stress and anxiety.

Stress and anxiety can have a negative influence on general health, and they are especially harmful for persons with chronic renal disease (CKD). Regular exercise can help to reduce stress and anxiety, which can benefit kidney function.

They can cause the release of stress hormones such as cortisol, which can be harmful to the body. Cortisol levels that are too high can raise blood pressure, raise glucose levels, and contribute to inflammation. This can place additional strain on the heart and blood vessels over time, raising the risk of heart disease and stroke.

Exercise has been shown to be an effective stress and anxiety reducer. When you exercise, your body produces endorphins, which are natural compounds that can help you feel less stressed and anxious. Furthermore, exercise can help relieve muscle tension and improve general mood, making it an excellent stress and anxiety management tool.

Aside from the immediate advantages of exercise for stress and anxiety reduction, regular exercise can also help build resilience over time. Making exercise a regular part of your routine can aid in the development of your general mental and physical resilience, making it simpler to manage stress and anxiety in the future.

It is critical to remember that exercise should be done in moderation and under the supervision of a healthcare expert. Some types of exercise, such as strenuous physical activity or contact sports, may not be suitable for those with CKD. Your healthcare provider may provide you with personalized advice on the type and frequency of exercise that is best for you, taking into account your personal health status as well as any other medical concerns you may have.

Juicing for Kidney Health

Finally, decreasing stress and anxiety is a vital part of maintaining kidney function. Exercise can help alleviate stress and anxiety by releasing endorphins and relaxing muscles. Furthermore, incorporating exercise into your daily routine can assist in building resilience, making it simpler to manage stress and anxiety in the future. Always consult with your healthcare professional before making significant changes to your exercise habits to ensure that the fitness program you choose is safe and appropriate for your unique health state.

Improved muscle strength and flexibility.

Muscle strength and flexibility are vital parts of overall health and well-being, and they can also help kidney health. Exercise can assist in increasing muscular strength and flexibility in a variety of ways, making it an important component of a complete approach to kidney health management.

Exercise promotes the creation of new muscle tissue and increases the size and strength of existing muscle fibers, which can aid in building muscle strength. When you exercise, your muscles have to work harder than they normally do, which might help you gain strength over time. Furthermore, exercise can assist in enhancing muscle endurance, allowing you to undertake physical tasks for longer periods of time without becoming weary.

Muscle strength can benefit kidney health in a variety of ways. Strong muscles, for example, can aid in supporting good posture and improving balance, lowering the risk of falls and accidents. Muscle strength can also help lower the risk of back pain, which is frequent in people with kidney disease. Furthermore, strong muscles can help increase overall mobility, making daily activities easier and lowering the chance of physical limitations.

Flexibility is a crucial part of general health and well-being, as well as promoting kidney health. The ability of your muscles and joints to move through their complete range of motion is referred to as "flexibility." When you have good flexibility, you are less likely to experience stiffness and discomfort, and you are also less likely to be injured.

Stretching the muscles and enhancing joint mobility can help to improve flexibility. Stretching exercises, for example, can help to alleviate muscular tension and enhance joint range of motion.

Juicing for Kidney Health

Stretching can also assist in lessening the likelihood of muscular imbalances, which can lead to joint pain and damage.

It is vital to remember that exercise should be done in moderation and under the supervision of a healthcare expert. Some types of exercise, such as strenuous physical activity or contact sports, may not be suitable for those with chronic kidney disease (CKD). Your healthcare provider may provide you with personalized advice on the type and frequency of exercise that is best for you, taking into account your personal health status as well as any other medical concerns you may have.

Finally, increased muscle strength and flexibility are vital parts of overall health and well-being, and they can also help with kidney health. Exercise can help to increase muscle strength, endurance, and flexibility and minimize the chance of injury. Always consult with your healthcare professional before making significant changes to your exercise habits to ensure that the fitness program you choose is safe and appropriate for your unique health state.

Better overall physical and mental well-being.

Exercise is well known for its numerous physical and mental health advantages, and it can also help with kidney health. Exercise can help to create greater overall physical and mental well-being, improve quality of life, and enhance long-term health when done on a regular basis.

Improved physical fitness is one of the most important advantages of exercise. Regular exercise can help to improve cardiovascular fitness, muscle strength, flexibility, and injury risko improve cardiovascular fitness, muscle strength, flexibility, and injury risk. All of these characteristics can assist in improving general physical health and lowering the risk of chronic diseases, including heart disease, diabetes, and some types of cancer.

Exercise, in addition to boosting physical health, can also improve mental health. Exercise has been demonstrated to alleviate stress, anxiety, and sadness while also improving mood and self-esteem. Endorphins, which are natural substances in the body that have a favorable influence on mood, are released during exercise. Furthermore, exercise can lower the risk of cognitive decline and memory loss, as well as improve cognitive function in older persons.

Juicing for Kidney Health

Exercise can be especially beneficial for people with chronic kidney disease (CKD). CKD can cause a variety of physical and mental health issues, as well as have a substantial influence on quality of life. Regular exercise can assist persons with CKD in improving their physical function, minimizing symptoms, and enhancing their overall well-being.

Exercise should be done in moderation and under the supervision of a healthcare expert. Some types of exercise, such as strenuous physical activity or contact sports, may not be suitable for those with CKD. Your healthcare provider may provide you with personalized advice on the type and frequency of exercise that is best for you, taking into account your personal health status as well as any other medical concerns you may have.

Finally, exercise can play an important role in improving overall physical and emotional well-being in patients with CKD. Exercise on a regular basis can enhance physical fitness, reduce stress and anxiety, and boost mood and self-esteem. As with other aspects of health and well-being, working with a healthcare practitioner to establish a safe and effective fitness program that takes your particular health status and any other medical concerns you may have into account is essential.

Types of Exercise for CKD Patients

Low-impact activities.

Physical activity is a crucial aspect of preserving general health and well-being for those with chronic kidney disease (CKD). Many types of exercise, however, such as vigorous physical activity or contact sports, may not be suitable for those with CKD. Low-impact activities can be an excellent way to encourage physical activity and support kidney function in certain situations.

Low-impact activities are workouts that put little strain on the joints, making them gentler on the body and lowering the chance of injury. Walking, swimming, cycling, and yoga are examples of these types of workouts that are appropriate for patients with CKD who may have restricted mobility or joint pain.

Walking is one of the most basic and widely available kinds of low-impact exercise. Walking can help you improve your cardiovascular health, endurance, and muscle strength. It can also aid in the reduction of stress and anxiety, as well as the improvement of mood and self-esteem. Walking can be done anywhere, at any time, and with no particular equipment.

Swimming is yet another low-impact sport that can be beneficial to those with CKD. Swimming is a total-body activity that can help enhance muscle strength and cardiovascular health. It is also an excellent form of exercise for people who have joint pain or mobility issues because the buoyancy of the water helps to relieve joint tension.

Cycling is yet another low-impact sport that can be beneficial to those with CKD. Cycling is an effective kind of cardiovascular exercise that can improve muscle strength and endurance and reduce the risk of heart disease. Cycling can be done on a stationary bike or outside on a conventional cycle.

Yoga is a type of exercise that incorporates physical activity as well as mindfulness and meditation. Yoga can enhance physical flexibility and muscle strength while also reducing stress, anxiety, and despair. Yoga can be done in a class or at home, and no special equipment is required.

All forms of exercise, including low-impact exercises, should be done in moderation and under the supervision of a healthcare expert. Your healthcare provider may provide you with personalized advice on the type and frequency of exercise that is best for you, taking into account your personal health status as well as any other medical concerns you may have.

Low-impact exercises can be a great way for people with CKD to promote physical activity while also supporting renal function. Walking, swimming, cycling, and yoga are all gentle on the body, lowering the risk of injury while also improving cardiovascular fitness and muscle strength and reducing stress and anxiety. As with other aspects of health and well-being, working with a healthcare practitioner to establish a safe and effective fitness program that takes your particular health status and any other medical concerns you may have into account is essential.

Resistance training.

Resistance training is an important type of exercise for people who have chronic kidney disease (CKD). Resistance training, often known as strength training, includes working the muscles with resistance such as weights or resistance bands. This form of exercise can help people with CKD improve their muscle strength, flexibility, and general physical and mental well-being.

It can be beneficial for people with CKD because it can help reduce the disease's progression. Muscle mass and strength can decrease when kidney function declines, resulting in diminished mobility and general physical function. Resistance training can assist in mitigating this by increasing muscle mass and strength, which improves general physical function and quality of life.

Furthermore, resistance exercise can improve cardiovascular health, which is vital for kidney function. Resistance exercise on a regular basis can assist in developing cardiovascular endurance, lowering blood pressure, and improving heart health. This is significant for those with CKD since cardiovascular illness is a prevalent consequence of the disease.

Individuals with CKD should consult with their healthcare physician to identify the best type and amount of resistance exercise for their specific needs. Resistance training can be done at a gym or at home with weights, resistance bands, or bodyweight exercises.

It is also critical to begin slowly and gradually increase the intensity and quantity of resistance training over time. This will help to prevent damage and ensure the individual's safe progression. Furthermore, it is critical to be hydrated before, during, and after weight training, especially for people with CKD.

Finally, it can be a significant form of exercise for those with CKD since it improves muscle strength, flexibility, cardiovascular health, and general physical and mental well-being. Working with a healthcare physician to determine the optimum type and amount of resistance training for the individual's needs is as critical as beginning slowly and progressively increasing the intensity over time.

Aerobic exercise.

Aerobic exercise, often known as cardiovascular exercise, is essential for those with chronic kidney disease (CKD). Aerobic exercise is defined as any activity that raises the heart rate and enhances cardiovascular fitness, such as brisk walking, cycling, swimming, or dancing. This

Juicing for Kidney Health

form of activity can assist people with CKD in improving their cardiovascular health, energy levels, and general physical and mental well-being.

It improves cardiovascular health by boosting the heart rate, which improves blood flow, lowers blood pressure, and improves heart health. This is significant for those with CKD since cardiovascular illness is a prevalent consequence of the disease. Aerobic activity can help to enhance circulation, which can aid in the removal of waste products from the body and overall renal function.

It can also assist in boosting energy levels, which can be especially beneficial for those with CKD who are weary or fatigued. Aerobic exercise on a regular basis can enhance general physical and mental well-being as well as reduce tension and worry.

Individuals with CKD should consult with their healthcare physician to establish the best type and amount of aerobic exercise for their specific needs. Aerobic exercise at a moderate level for 30 minutes, three to four times a week, is recommended. Low-impact activities, such as walking or cycling, are frequently recommended for people with CKD because they place less strain on the kidneys and other organs.

Starting softly and progressively increasing the intensity and duration of aerobic exercise over time is also helpful. This will help to prevent damage and ensure the individual's safe progression. Furthermore, it is critical to be hydrated before, during, and after aerobic exercise, especially for people with CKD.

In summary, aerobic exercise is an important form of exercise for people with CKD since it provides a variety of benefits such as improved cardiovascular health, enhanced energy levels, and general physical and mental well-being. Working with a healthcare physician to determine the optimum type and amount of aerobic exercise for the individual's needs is as critical as beginning slowly and progressively increasing the intensity over time.

Stretching and yoga.

Stretching and yoga are two types of exercise that can benefit people with chronic kidney disease (CKD). Stretching and yoga can both assist in increasing flexibility, decreasing stress and anxiety, and promoting general physical and mental well-being.

Juicing for Kidney Health

Stretching exercises entail holding a specific position for a given amount of time in order to build flexibility and range of motion. These exercises can help to alleviate muscle stress and soreness while also improving circulation, which is important for those with CKD. Stretching exercises can also help you improve your balance and coordination, which can help you avoid falls and injuries.

Yoga is a workout that incorporates physical postures, breathing methods, and meditation. It can aid with flexibility, strength, and balance, as well as stress and anxiety reduction. Yoga can also assist in improving circulation, which is important for those with CKD, as well as overall physical and emotional well-being.

Individuals with CKD should consult with their healthcare provider to determine the type and amount of stretching and yoga activities that are appropriate for their specific needs.Low-impact stretching and yoga exercises are frequently recommended for people with CKD because they place less strain on the kidneys and other organs.

Stretching and yoga exercises should be started cautiously and gradually increased in intensity and duration over time. This will help to prevent damage and ensure the individual's safe progression. Furthermore, it is critical to be hydrated before, during, and after stretching and yoga sessions, especially for people with CKD.

They are types of exercise that can benefit people with CKD by improving flexibility, reducing stress and anxiety, and improving overall physical and mental well-being. Working with a healthcare physician to determine the optimum type and amount of stretching and yoga exercises for the individual's needs is critical, as is beginning slowly and progressively increasing the intensity over time.

Conclusion

Summary of the benefits of exercise and hydration.

Exercise and hydration are crucial components of a healthy lifestyle, and they provide several benefits for those with and without chronic kidney disease (CKD).

Juicing for Kidney Health

Physical activity has been found to promote cardiovascular health by lowering the risk of heart disease and stroke. It can also assist to preserve renal function and lower the risk of kidney injury by improving circulation. Exercise has also been demonstrated to lower stress and anxiety, increase muscle strength and flexibility, and contribute to general physical and mental well-being.

Low-impact activities, such as walking or cycling, are appropriate choices for people with CKD because they place less strain on the kidneys and other organs. Resistance training, such as weightlifting, can also aid to maintain overall health by improving muscle strength. Running or swimming, for example, can help to enhance cardiovascular health and overall fitness. Stretching and yoga can help with flexibility and stress reduction.

Individuals with CKD should speak with a healthcare physician before beginning an exercise program, since the provider can advise on what types of exercise are appropriate and what to avoid. It is also critical to begin slowly and progressively increase the intensity and length of exercise over time.

Hydration is particularly crucial for those with CKD because it helps to remove waste and extra fluid from the body, lowering the risk of kidney damage. Other drinks may include excessive quantities of sugar, salt, or other compounds that can affect the kidneys, therefore drinking water is the greatest option for hydration. Individuals with CKD should speak with a healthcare specialist to establish how much water they should drink each day, as this varies based on the individual's health status and illness stage.

In summary, exercise and hydration are essential components of a healthy lifestyle, and they have various benefits for those with CKD. Individuals with CKD should check with a healthcare physician before beginning an activity program and determining their daily water needs. Exercise and hydration can assist improve cardiovascular health, lower stress and anxiety, increase muscle strength and flexibility, and contribute to overall physical and mental well-being.

Juicing for Kidney Health

Importance of incorporating exercise and hydration into a comprehensive approach to managing CKD.

It is impossible to overestimate the importance of including exercise and hydration in a holistic strategy for controlling chronic kidney disease (CKD). Exercise and hydration are important in sustaining kidney health and enhancing CKD patients' overall quality of life.

Exercise provides several health benefits for the kidneys. It contributes to better cardiovascular health by lowering the risk of heart disease, a frequent consequence of CKD. Exercise also improves circulation, which is beneficial to kidney health because the kidneys rely on adequate blood flow to operate properly. Exercise can also assist in increasing muscle strength and flexibility, lowering the risk of falls and fractures in the elderly. Exercise has also been demonstrated to lower tension and anxiety as well as increase general physical and mental well-being.

Walking, cycling, and swimming are excellent low-impact exercises for CKD patients. These exercises are easy on the joints and can be done for extended periods of time without causing undue pressure on the body. Resistance training, such as weightlifting, can also be useful for CKD patients if done correctly and under the guidance of a healthcare expert. Aerobic exercise, such as running or jumping rope, is another excellent alternative for CKD patients since it enhances cardiovascular health and overall fitness. Stretching and yoga are also excellent choices for CKD patients since they can improve flexibility, balance, and posture.

We should also mention that exercise can aid in enhancing hydration levels because it raises the body's requirement for liquids. Hydration is essential for kidney health because it aids in the removal of waste and toxins from the body. Furthermore, hydration is critical for maintaining normal blood pressure, which is critical for kidney function because high blood pressure is a major consequence of CKD.

In summary, exercise and hydration are critical components of a comprehensive CKD management strategy. Before beginning any new exercise program, CKD patients should talk with their healthcare professional, since the type and intensity of exercise may need to be altered based on their specific health state and kidney function. Patients' general health, well-being, and

Juicing for Kidney Health

quality of life can be improved by including exercise and hydration in a comprehensive strategy for controlling CKD.

Final thoughts on the role of exercise and hydration in supporting kidney health.

Exercise and hydration are essential for those with chronic kidney disease (CKD) to maintain kidney health. A holistic approach to controlling CKD and fostering general well-being must include regular physical exercise and sufficient hydration.

Physical activity improves cardiovascular health, circulation, and muscle strength while also lowering stress and anxiety. Aerobic exercise, weight training, stretching and yoga, and low-impact activities are all sorts of physical activity that are good for people with CKD. Before beginning a new fitness program, it is critical to select exercises that are appropriate for your unique needs and limits and to check with a healthcare specialist.

Adequate hydration is also important for kidney health since it aids in the removal of waste and toxins from the body, as well as the regulation of blood pressure and the maintenance of optimal fluid levels. The recommended daily fluid intake for people with CKD varies based on their specific condition and treatment plan, so consult with your doctor to find out what is best for you.

The importance of including exercise and hydration in a holistic approach to CKD management cannot be overemphasized. Regular physical exercise and regular hydration can enhance overall physical and mental well-being as well as kidney health by lowering the risk of additional injury and boosting treatment effectiveness.

Exercise and hydration are critical components of a holistic strategy to CKD management, and people with CKD should consult with a healthcare physician to establish the best method for their specific needs and limits. Regular physical exercise and sufficient hydration should be incorporated into your daily routine to support kidney function, improve overall well-being, and promote a healthy lifestyle.

Juicing for Kidney Health

CHAPTER 12

Understanding Medication and Supplements for Kidney Health

Overview of the importance of medication and supplements in managing kidney health.

In people with chronic kidney disease (CKD), medications and supplements are critical for maintaining renal health. CKD is a progressive illness that impairs the kidneys' ability to filter waste from the blood. If neglected, it can progress to end-stage renal disease (ESRD), necessitating dialysis or a kidney transplant.

To help control the symptoms of CKD and limit its progression, medications and nutrients are administered. They can aid in the control of excessive blood pressure, the reduction of cholesterol, and the regulation of mineral and electrolyte levels in the body. Medications can also help treat anemia, a common consequence of CKD, by enhancing red blood cell production.

Vitamin D and calcium supplements, for example, can help prevent bone disease, which is another major complication of CKD. They can also aid in the maintenance of overall health and well-being.

It should be noted that not all drugs and supplements are appropriate for people with CKD. Some can have negative side effects, interact with other medications, or worsen kidney conditions. Working closely with a healthcare physician to establish which medications and supplements are safe and appropriate for each individual is critical.

In conclusion, drugs and supplements play a significant role in the management of renal health in people with CKD. They can help manage symptoms, halt disease progression, and prevent or manage consequences. However, it is critical to get the advice of a healthcare expert to ensure that they are safe and appropriate for each individual.

Juicing for Kidney Health

Medications and supplements play a significant role in the treatment and maintenance of renal health. Medication can be used to manage symptoms, reduce the progression of the disease, and control related problems in people with chronic kidney disease (CKD).

Certain drugs, for example, can be used to treat high blood pressure, a common and significant consequence of CKD. High blood pressure can harm the blood vessels in the kidneys, causing renal function to deteriorate further. Medication that controls blood pressure can help preserve renal function and lower the chance of kidney failure.

Medications can also be used to treat high blood levels of waste products like creatinine and urea. When the kidneys aren't working properly, waste products build up and create symptoms including weariness, nausea, and muscle cramps. Medication can assist in improving overall well-being and reducing the risk of problems by lowering the levels of these waste products.

Supplements, in addition to pharmaceuticals, can play a significant role in renal health management. Individuals with CKD, for example, may require more vitamins and minerals, such as iron and vitamin D, to compensate for losses owing to impaired renal function. They may also require supplements to maintain electrolyte balance and treat symptoms such as anemia.

It is important to note that medications and supplements might have negative effects and interact with other pharmaceuticals, so working with a healthcare provider to carefully manage and monitor these therapies is essential. A healthcare practitioner can also assist in determining the appropriate type and dosage of drugs and supplements to match a person's specific needs and goals.

In conclusion, drugs and supplements are critical for maintaining kidney health and treating renal illness. They can help regulate symptoms, halt disease development, and lower the risk of complications. It is, however, critical to collaborate with a healthcare expert to ensure that these treatments are utilized safely and efficiently.

Juicing for Kidney Health

Importance of working with a healthcare provider to manage medications and supplements.

When it comes to managing drugs and supplements for kidney health, working with a healthcare provider is vital. This is due to a number of factors, including:

1. Individualized care: Everyone's kidney health is different, and their treatment plan should reflect that. When deciding the appropriate course of therapy, a healthcare provider will consider criteria such as age, overall health, and the precise type and stage of kidney disease.

2.Monitoring side effects: Some drugs and supplements can have side effects that affect the kidneys or other organs. A healthcare professional will keep an eye out for these adverse effects and modify the treatment plan as necessary.

3. Determining proper dosages: The correct dosage of a medication or supplement depends on the individual. A healthcare provider will assist you in determining the appropriate dose depending on characteristics such as age, weight, and the existence of other medical conditions.

4.Avoiding interactions: Some drugs and supplements can have negative interactions. These interactions will be identified by a healthcare provider, and the treatment plan will be adjusted accordingly.

Kidney illness therapy is always evolving, and a healthcare provider will be able to stay current on the latest improvements in drug and supplement treatments.

Working with a healthcare physician to manage drugs and supplements for kidney health is critical. A healthcare provider may personalize the treatment plan, monitor for side effects, identify optimum dosages, avoid interactions, and keep current on advances in kidney disease treatment.

Juicing for Kidney Health

Medications for Kidney Disease

Overview of common medications used in treating kidney disease.

Medication plays an important role in the therapy of kidney disease by decreasing the course of the disease and alleviating symptoms. Here are some of the most commonly used drugs for treating renal disease:

1. **Angiotensin-Converting Enzyme (ACE) Inhibitors:** These drugs lower blood pressure and reduce kidney stress. They function by inhibiting the synthesis of a hormone that constricts blood vessels and raises blood pressure.

2.**Angiotensin II Receptor Blockers (ARBs):** ARBs, like ACE inhibitors, serve to lower blood pressure and minimize kidney stress. They function by inhibiting the action of a hormone that constricts blood vessels and raises blood pressure.

3. **Anti-inflammatory medications:** Nonsteroidal anti-inflammatory drugs (NSAIDs) such as ibuprofen, naproxen, and aspirin can promote renal inflammation and be detrimental to the kidneys. As a result, patients with kidney illness should avoid these medications or use them only under the supervision of a healthcare expert.

4. **Diuretics:** These medications aid in the removal of excess fluid from the body and the reduction of edema. They are most typically used to treat hypertension and heart failure, but they can also be used to treat kidney illness.

5. **Vitamin D supplements:** People with renal illness may need to take vitamin D supplements to keep their bones strong because their kidneys may not manufacture enough of this vitamin on their own.

6.**Iron supplements:** People with renal illness may require iron supplements as a result of anemia caused by red blood cell loss.

It is important to remember that not all drugs and supplements are appropriate for everyone and that you should consult with a healthcare expert to establish what is best for your specific requirements. This could mean altering dosages, switching drugs, or avoiding certain supplements entirely.

Juicing for Kidney Health

A mix of drugs and nutrients is frequently used to delay the progression of kidney disease, treat symptoms, and preserve general health. People with kidney illnesses can ensure that they are taking the appropriate drugs and supplements by working closely with their healthcare professional.

Angiotensin-converting enzyme inhibitors (ACE inhibitors) and angiotensin receptor blockers (ARBs).

Angiotensin-converting enzyme inhibitors (ACE inhibitors) and angiotensin receptor blockers (ARBs) are two drugs that are routinely used to treat renal disease. They are both medication types used to treat high blood pressure and enhance kidney function.

ACE inhibitors function by preventing the synthesis of angiotensin II, a hormone that constricts blood vessels and raises blood pressure. This relaxes the blood vessels, allowing blood to flow more freely and relieving stress on the heart and kidneys. ACE inhibitors also prevent the body from manufacturing aldosterone, a hormone that causes the kidneys to retain salt and fluid, resulting in fluid accumulation and swelling.

ARBs, on the other hand, work by inhibiting angiotensin II from attaching to its receptors in the blood vessels. The same blood pressure-lowering and blood vessel-dilating actions as ACE inhibitors are achieved.

In individuals with chronic kidney disease (CKD) and diabetic nephropathy, both ACE inhibitors and ARBs have been demonstrated to improve kidney function and decrease the course of kidney disease. They can also aid in the reduction of proteinuria, or the presence of excess protein in the urine, which is a common sign of kidney impairment.

Some individuals may experience side effects such as coughing, dizziness, headache, and impaired kidney function as a result of these drugs. As a result, working with a healthcare practitioner to monitor the effects of these medications and change the dose as needed is critical.

In conclusion, ACE inhibitors and ARBs are critical in the management of renal disease and the improvement of kidney function. They should only be used under the supervision and advice of a healthcare provider.

Juicing for Kidney Health

Diuretics.

Diuretics are drugs that increase urine flow to help the body clear itself of excess fluid. They are essential in the treatment of renal illness because they help to relieve fluid buildup, lower blood pressure, and minimize the strain on the heart and kidneys. Diuretics are often used to treat illnesses such as edema (swelling caused by an excess of fluid) and hypertension (high blood pressure).

They are classified into three types: loop diuretics, thiazide diuretics, and potassium-sparing diuretics. The strongest loop diuretics, such as furosemide, are commonly used to treat severe edema or heart failure. Hydrochlorothiazide and other thiazide diuretics are routinely used to treat hypertension and mild to moderate edema. Spironolactone and other potassium-sparing diuretics are used to treat hypertension and edema while simultaneously maintaining potassium levels in the body.

Remember that diuretics can cause electrolyte imbalances, dehydration, and muscle cramps. Furthermore, they may interfere with other medications and supplements, so it is critical to consult with a healthcare expert before using them. While using diuretics, it is also vital to assess kidney function, electrolyte levels, and blood pressure on a regular basis.

In summary, diuretics are important in the therapy of renal disease because they help to relieve fluid buildup, lower blood pressure, and minimize the strain on the heart and kidneys. However, it is critical to collaborate with a healthcare provider to ensure that they are used safely and effectively.

Calcium channel blockers.

Calcium channel blockers, also known as calcium antagonists, are a class of medication used to treat hypertension, or high blood pressure, which is a common complication of chronic kidney disease (CKD). Calcium channel blockers function by preventing calcium ions from entering the cells of the heart and blood vessels. These drugs help to relax the blood vessels, which can lower

Juicing for Kidney Health

blood pressure and reduce the burden on the heart by reducing the amount of calcium entering these cells.

High blood pressure is a critical contributor to the advancement of renal disease in people with CKD. Calcium channel blockers can help halt the progression of renal disease and lower the risk of future problems by managing blood pressure. Calcium channel blockers can also be used to treat other CKD problems, like heart disease and peripheral artery disease.

Calcium channel blockers are typically given orally once or twice daily. Calcium channel blockers often used include amlodipine, nifedipine, and diltiazem. Calcium channel blockers may interfere with other drugs and supplements; therefore, it is critical to consult with a healthcare provider to monitor their use.

Finally, calcium channel blockers have a significant role in the treatment of hypertension and other CKD consequences. These drugs help lower blood pressure, relieve heart strain, and slow the progression of renal disease. Individuals with CKD can safely add calcium channel blockers to their treatment plan and achieve better overall kidney health by consulting with a healthcare specialist.

Phosphorus binders.

Phosphorus binders are drugs used to help regulate high phosphorus levels in the blood, which are frequent in people with kidney disease. Phosphorus is a vital mineral found in a variety of foods, including dairy, meat, and some grains. In healthy people, the kidneys filter out extra phosphorus and maintain normal levels. When the kidneys are not functioning properly, as is the situation with kidney disease, they are unable to adequately eliminate excess phosphorus, resulting in increased amounts in the blood.

Elevated phosphorus levels can lead to a variety of concerns, including soft tissue calcification, an increased risk of cardiovascular disease, and osteoporosis. Phosphorus binders are frequently prescribed by healthcare practitioners to treat these concerns. Phosphorus binders inhibit phosphorus absorption into the bloodstream by adhering to it in the gastrointestinal system. This reduces blood phosphorus levels and the risk of linked health concerns.

Juicing for Kidney Health

They are classified into three types: calcium-based binders, non-calcium-based binders, and combination binders. Calcium-based binders, such as calcium carbonate, function by creating a compound in the gut with phosphorus that is not taken into the bloodstream. Non-calcium-based binders, such as sevelamer, bind to phosphorus in a similar fashion but do not include calcium, which can be advantageous for people who have high calcium levels in their blood. Lanthanum carbonate, for example, contains both calcium and a non-calcium-based binder.

Phosphorus binders should be taken with meals rather than on their own, as they will not operate well without food. Working with a healthcare physician to identify the optimum dose of phosphorus binders is also vital, as is monitoring blood phosphorus levels to ensure that they are adequately managed.

In conclusion, phosphorus binders play a vital role in regulating high phosphorus levels in the blood in persons with kidney disease. They function by binding to phosphorus in the gastrointestinal tract and inhibiting its absorption into the circulation, so lowering blood phosphorus levels and lowering the risk of associated health problems. However, working with a healthcare physician to identify the proper dose and monitor blood phosphorus levels is critical to ensuring that they are adequately maintained.

Vitamin D and iron supplements.

Vitamin D and iron are crucial minerals for overall health, and people with chronic kidney disease (CKD) may require additional supplementation to keep their levels acceptable.

It is necessary for bone health because it aids in calcium absorption. People with CKD, on the other hand, are frequently unable to make enough vitamin D because the kidneys are in charge of converting it into its active form. As a result, they may need to take vitamin D supplements to avoid vitamin D insufficiency, which can lead to osteoporosis.

Iron is a component of hemoglobin, which transports oxygen in the blood. Anemia, which can be caused by a shortage of iron in the body, is common in people with CKD. Iron supplements may be required to maintain healthy levels and aid in the treatment of anemia.

Juicing for Kidney Health

Working with a healthcare physician to identify the optimum dose of vitamin D and iron supplements is critical since excessive supplementation can impair kidney function. A healthcare provider can also keep an eye out for any negative side effects and modify dosages as needed.

Supplementing with vitamin D and iron as part of a holistic strategy for CKD management can help enhance overall health and support renal function.

Supplements for Kidney Health

Overview of commonly used supplements.

Supplements can help maintain kidney health, but it's vital to talk to your doctor before starting any supplement routine. Omega-3 fatty acids, magnesium, and probiotics are among the prominent kidney health supplements.

Fish oil contains omega-3 fatty acids, which can aid in reducing inflammation, controlling blood pressure, and enhancing kidney function. Furthermore, magnesium supplements may help patients with chronic kidney disease (CKD) maintain adequate magnesium levels, as CKD can lead to a magnesium deficit. Probiotics may also benefit kidney function by promoting a healthy gut flora, which has an impact on general health and well-being.

Note that supplements should not be utilized in place of a well-balanced diet. They should be combined with a diet high in fruits and vegetables, lean protein, and healthy fats. Furthermore, it is critical to inform your healthcare professional about all supplements you are taking, as some may interfere with drugs or impair kidney function.

Supplements can be a beneficial addition to a holistic approach to kidney health management, but they must be used in conjunction with a healthcare provider to ensure that they are taken safely and efficiently.

Juicing for Kidney Health

Omega-3 fatty acids.

Omega-3 fatty acids are a form of polyunsaturated fat that is necessary for human health. These fatty acids are essential for a variety of body processes, including inflammation reduction, heart health promotion, and brain function support.

They have been demonstrated to provide a range of benefits in the context of renal health. Some research has found that omega-3 fatty acids can help reduce inflammation in people with chronic kidney disease (CKD). Because inflammation contributes to the progression of kidney disease, lowering it can help reduce the illness's progression.

Furthermore, they have been demonstrated to promote cardiovascular health, which is significant for people with CKD because they are predisposed to heart disease. This is because waste product accumulation in the blood, which is frequent in patients with CKD, can damage blood vessels, raising the risk of cardiovascular disease.

Omega-3 fatty acids are also necessary for good renal function. They have been found, for example, to help manage blood pressure, which is important for people with CKD because uncontrolled high blood pressure can further damage the kidneys.

These acids are most typically encountered in the form of fish oil in supplements. Fish oil supplements are widely available and simple to add to a nutritious diet. However, not all fish oil supplements are made equal, and some may include impurities, so choosing a high-quality, purified fish oil supplement that has been tested for purity and potency is critical.

In conclusion, omega-3 fatty acids are a useful supplement for persons with renal disease since they can help reduce inflammation, enhance cardiovascular health, and keep kidney function good. Before beginning a new supplement regimen, like with all supplements, consult with a healthcare provider to ensure that it is safe and appropriate for you.

Magnesium.

Magnesium is an essential mineral that the body requires for a variety of tasks. It is essential for preserving bone, heart, and kidney function. According to research, magnesium may be advantageous to kidney function, particularly in people with chronic kidney disease (CKD).

Juicing for Kidney Health

Magnesium levels in CKD patients might become unbalanced, resulting in hypomagnesemia. This syndrome is linked to a variety of health issues, such as heart disease, osteoporosis, and high blood pressure. Magnesium supplements may assist in restoring this imbalance and improving general health.

Magnesium supplementation has been found in studies to help lessen the chance of getting kidney stones. It may also help enhance insulin sensitivity and lower blood pressure, both of which are significant variables in maintaining kidney health sensitivity and lower blood pressure, both of which are significant variables in maintaining kidney health. Magnesium has also been demonstrated to delay the course of CKD, potentially decreasing the decline in renal function.

Magnesium is crucial for general health and wellness, in addition to its potential benefits for kidney health. It is involved in nearly 300 various metabolic activities in the body, including glucose, protein, and fat metabolism. It also aids in the maintenance of healthy bones, the regulation of heart rhythm, and the support of the immune system.

It is critical to consult a healthcare physician when considering magnesium supplements to establish the optimum dose. Excessive magnesium consumption can cause diarrhea, nausea, and abdominal cramping. Individuals with CKD should have their renal function constantly checked, as magnesium levels in the blood can accumulate and cause additional health concerns.

Finally, magnesium is an important vitamin for sustaining kidney health and general wellness. Incorporating magnesium-rich foods or supplements into your diet may support kidney function, reduce your risk of developing kidney stones, and enhance your general health. However, it is critical to collaborate closely with a healthcare physician to identify the proper dose and monitor kidney function.

Vitamin C

Vitamin C, commonly known as ascorbic acid, is an essential nutrient that is required for numerous bodily activities, including the formation and maintenance of healthy skin, bones, and connective tissue, as well as collagen production and iron absorption. Furthermore, vitamin C is

Juicing for Kidney Health

an antioxidant that helps prevent cells from being damaged by free radicals, which can lead to chronic diseases like cancer and heart disease.

It can be very beneficial to those with renal disease in terms of overall health and well-being. This is because renal illness can impede the body's ability to manufacture and store vitamin C, as well as affect the body's ability to eliminate excess vitamin C. As a result, persons with renal illness may be at risk for vitamin C insufficiency, which can cause anemia, lethargy, and a weaker immune system, among other things.

To maintain appropriate vitamin C consumption, persons with renal disease should eat a balanced diet that includes vitamin C-rich foods such as citrus fruits, berries, leafy greens, and peppers. Taking a vitamin C supplement under the supervision of a healthcare professional may also be beneficial for certain people with kidney disease, especially if they have a deficiency or are unable to meet their vitamin C needs through diet alone.

Too much vitamin C can be dangerous to people with renal disease because it can cause kidney stones, increase oxidative stress, and interfere with the efficacy of some treatments. As a result, it is critical to collaborate with a healthcare professional to determine the appropriate vitamin C dose for your specific needs and to track your vitamin C levels over time.

Finally, vitamin C is a crucial component for persons with renal disease, and adopting a balanced diet and the appropriate supplement regimen under the supervision of a healthcare provider can help support general health and well-being.

Probiotics.

Probiotics are dietary supplements containing live bacteria or yeast that are meant to promote healthy gut flora. They are gaining popularity as a supplement for a variety of health concerns, including kidney health. While the precise effects of probiotics on the kidney are unknown, some research suggests that probiotics may enhance renal function in certain circumstances.

According to one study, individuals with chronic kidney disease (CKD) who took a probiotic supplement had better renal function, less inflammation, and less oxidative stress than those who did not take the supplement. Another study discovered that probiotics enhanced gastrointestinal function in CKD patients, which improved the absorption of critical nutrients required for healthy kidney functioning.

Probiotics have been demonstrated to have numerous health benefits, such as enhanced digestive health, lower inflammation, and increased immunological function, in addition to their potential benefits for kidney health. This is due to the importance of the gut microbiome in overall health and well-being.

Although they may have some benefits for kidney health, they should not be taken in place of established medical therapies. People with renal disease should always consult with their doctor to identify the best strategy to manage their condition.

Furthermore, not all probiotics are created equal, and some may be better for kidney health than others. It is critical to choose high-quality supplements that have been evaluated for purity, potency, and efficacy and to adhere to the label's recommended dosage. People with kidney disease should also be cautious about selecting probiotics that are appropriate for their condition and discussing their use with their doctor.

Herbs and plant extracts.

Herbs and plant extracts have been utilized as traditional treatments for a variety of health concerns for ages. Some herbs and plant extracts have been examined for their potential advantages in the context of renal health. However, it should be noted that the use of herbs and plant extracts should always be done under the supervision of a healthcare professional.

Herbs and plant extracts that are often utilized for kidney health include:

Cranberry extract is often used to maintain urinary tract health because it may aid in the prevention of bacteria sticking to the urinary tract walls. It may possibly have antioxidant and anti-inflammatory properties that can benefit kidney function.

Nettle: Nettle is a herb known for its diuretic effects, as it can enhance urine flow and promote kidney function. It may possibly have anti-inflammatory properties and aid in the reduction of oxidative stress.

Juicing for Kidney Health

Turmeric: Turmeric is a spice that is often used in cooking and has been used as a traditional cure for a variety of health concerns for millennia. It contains a lot of antioxidants and has anti-inflammatory qualities, so it can aid in kidney health.

Milk thistle is an herb that is widely used to promote liver health. It contains a lot of antioxidants and may protect the kidneys from oxidative stress and inflammation.

Dandelion: For generations, dandelion has been used as a traditional medicine for a variety of health concerns, including kidney and liver health. It is a natural diuretic that may aid in the promotion of kidney function and fluid balance.

It's crucial to remember that not all herbs and plant extracts have been thoroughly researched for safety and efficacy, and some may interact with drugs or have other potential negative effects. It is always important to talk with a healthcare provider before consuming any herbs or plant extracts.

Choosing the Right Medications and Supplements

Factors to consider when choosing medications and supplements.

When selecting drugs and supplements for kidney health, numerous things should be considered. To begin, it is critical to collaborate with a healthcare provider to ensure that any medications or supplements are safe and appropriate for the individual's specific health needs and medical history. Because some drugs and supplements may interact with other prescriptions or have potentially serious side effects, it is critical to have a healthcare expert supervise and monitor their use.

Furthermore, when selecting drugs and supplements, it is critical to consider the kind and stage of kidney disease. Individuals with early-stage kidney disease, for example, may benefit more from drugs for high blood pressure or diabetes management, but those with severe kidney disease may require extra medications or supplements to manage symptoms or slow the advancement of their condition.

It is important to evaluate the dosage and frequency with which medications and supplements are taken, as well as any potential side effects or interactions with other medications or supplements.

Juicing for Kidney Health

Some drugs and supplements may necessitate regular blood testing or monitoring to ensure that they are being taken safely and efficiently.

Finally, consumers should be aware of the potential advantages and hazards of any medications or supplements and should seek additional information from their healthcare professional if they have any questions or concerns. In general, including a balanced diet and regular exercise in a holistic strategy to managing kidney illness, together with any necessary drugs or supplements, is frequently the best method to maintain overall kidney health.

Importance of dosage and frequency.

Those with chronic kidney disease (CKD), medications and supplements are critical in regulating renal health. The amount and frequency with which drugs and supplements for kidney health are used are important considerations.

Medication and supplement dosage and frequency are critical for maintaining optimal effectiveness while minimizing potential negative effects. The optimal dosage will be determined by several factors, including the individual's age, weight, medical history, and the severity of their renal disease.

For example, if someone is using a phosphorus binder, the dosage may need to be modified as their phosphorus levels fluctuate. Similarly, if a person takes vitamin D supplements, the dosage may need to be modified based on their vitamin D blood levels.

Certain medications and supplements may be harmful to the kidneys if taken in excess.This is why it is critical to collaborate with a healthcare provider to identify the appropriate dosage and frequency of use for each individual's unique requirements.

Always follow the instructions on the drug label, and never modify the dosage without first consulting a healthcare expert. It is critical to take drugs and supplements at the proper time and in the right doses to ensure their effectiveness in maintaining kidney health.

In conclusion, when selecting drugs and supplements for kidney health, the dosage and frequency of usage are critical elements to consider. Working with a healthcare professional to

Juicing for Kidney Health

identify the optimal dosage and frequency for each individual's special needs is critical, as is always following the recommendations on the medicine label.

Interactions between medications and supplements.

When managing kidney health, it is critical to evaluate not only the medications and supplements you are taking but also how they interact with one another. This is because some drugs and supplements can have detrimental effects on the kidneys and interact in potentially hazardous ways.

The possibility of increased risk of kidney injury is a typical interaction between drugs and supplements. Nonsteroidal anti-inflammatory medicines (NSAIDs) and magnesium supplements, for example, can raise the risk of kidney injury.

Furthermore, some supplements can interfere with drugs, reducing their effectiveness. Taking vitamin C alongside some drugs, such as iron supplements, can, for example, limit iron absorption.

When taking kidney-healthy drugs and supplements, it is critical to consult with a healthcare expert. A healthcare professional can assist you in determining the optimum medicine and supplement combination for your specific needs, as well as monitor any potential interactions between the medications and supplements you are taking.

It is also critical to inform your doctor if you are taking any supplements or herbs, as these may interact with your prescriptions or have unanticipated effects on your kidney health.

Finally, when maintaining kidney health, it is critical to evaluate the interactions between drugs and supplements. You can ensure that the drugs and supplements you are taking are safe and helpful for maintaining your kidney health by consulting with a healthcare professional and being aware of potential interactions.

Juicing for Kidney Health

Kidney disease management can be a complex procedure that necessitates a multifaceted strategy that involves medicine, vitamins, and lifestyle changes. When it comes to medication and supplements, it is critical for people with kidney disease to consider their bodies' specific demands as well as the impact that these goods may have on their overall health.

Individuals with renal disease may experience impaired kidney function, which can lead to a variety of health problems. As a result, selecting drugs and supplements that are especially developed to promote kidney function is critical. In general, drugs used to treat kidney disease are intended to help manage blood pressure, minimize proteinuria, and lower the risk of renal disease complications.

Angiotensin-converting enzyme inhibitors (ACE inhibitors), angiotensin receptor blockers (ARBs), diuretics, calcium channel blockers, and phosphorus binders are some popular drugs used to treat renal disease. Each of these medications has a distinct purpose in supporting kidney function, and it is critical to examine the potential benefits and dangers with a healthcare provider.

When it comes to vitamins, it is vital to select those that are specifically developed to promote kidney health. Omega-3 fatty acids, magnesium, vitamin C, probiotics, and herbs and plant extracts are some of the most commonly utilized supplements. However, it is critical to evaluate potential drug-supplement interactions as well as the optimal dosage and frequency of administration.

Finally, including drugs and supplements in a complete approach to controlling renal disease is critical for those suffering from this ailment. Individuals with kidney illnesses can improve their overall health and well-being by working with a healthcare professional and considering issues such as dosage, frequency, and potential interactions.

Juicing for Kidney Health

Importance of regularly monitoring medications and supplements.

Regular medication and supplement monitoring is critical for those with renal illness since the kidneys filter waste and excess chemicals from the body. Toxins can build up in the kidneys if they are not functioning properly, causing major health concerns.

The amount and frequency of drugs and supplements are two of the most significant factors to consider when managing them. To avoid unpleasant reactions and achieve the greatest outcomes for kidney health, it is critical to take drugs and supplements as advised by a healthcare expert.

In some situations, drugs and supplements can interact, resulting in unexpected or unwanted side effects. As a result, it is critical to keep track of all drugs and supplements used and to notify a healthcare professional of any modifications to the regimen.

It is good to perform routine blood and urine tests to assess kidney function. These tests can detect changes in kidney function and allow a doctor to alter drugs and supplements as necessary.

Furthermore, any negative effects that may occur when using drugs or supplements must be considered. If side effects develop, notify your healthcare practitioner immediately since they may need to alter the dosage or switch to a different drug or supplement.

Finally, people with kidney disease should check their prescriptions and supplements on a regular basis. It is critical to take medications and supplements as indicated, to be aware of potential interactions, and to assess kidney function and adverse effects on a frequent basis. Individuals can help to maximize their kidney health and avoid further difficulties by doing so.

Regular check-ins with healthcare providers.

Individuals with renal illness who are taking drugs and supplements must have regular check-ins with their healthcare professionals. A healthcare professional will evaluate the patient's condition, review any changes in their health status, and make any required adjustments to their medication and supplement regimen during these appointments. This ensures that the patient's drugs and supplements are performing properly and are not producing any side effects.

Juicing for Kidney Health

Regular check-ins have the added benefit of allowing healthcare providers to identify and resolve any concerns that may arise as a result of taking drugs and supplements. For example, if a patient has any side effects or the medications are not producing the expected outcomes, the healthcare professional can change the dosage, switch to a different prescription, or offer alternative treatment options.

It's also worth noting that when kidney disease advances, patients' prescriptions and supplements may need to be adjusted on a regular basis. Patients can guarantee that they are receiving the most suitable and effective therapies for their specific requirements by collaborating with a healthcare professional.

Monitoring kidney function is another crucial reason for regular check-ins with healthcare practitioners. Renal disease can cause changes in kidney function, which might affect the efficacy of drugs and supplements. Healthcare providers will monitor kidney function using blood tests and other diagnostic tools and will alter drugs and supplements as needed to support the patient's renal health.

Finally, regular check-ins with healthcare specialists are essential for those with renal disease who are taking medications and supplements. They allow patients to receive the most appropriate and effective therapies while also ensuring that their drugs and supplements are working properly and are not creating any bad reactions.

Side effects and potential reactions.

Although medications and supplements can help promote kidney health, they can also have side effects and adverse reactions. These adverse effects can range from moderate and controllable to severe and life-threatening, and it is critical that you are aware of them.

Common adverse effects of drugs for renal disease include nausea, dizziness, headaches, and weariness. ARBs and ACE inhibitors can produce a chronic cough, while diuretics can create an electrolyte imbalance, resulting in low potassium levels, which can cause muscle weakness, cramps, and irregular heartbeats. Calcium channel blockers can cause diarrhea, leg and ankle edema, and heart rate abnormalities.

Juicing for Kidney Health

Supplements including omega-3 fatty acids, magnesium, vitamin C, probiotics, and herbs and plant extracts can all have negative side effects. For example, omega-3 fatty acids, especially in large amounts, can increase the risk of bleeding. Magnesium supplements can produce diarrhea, nausea, and stomach cramps, and high vitamin C doses can cause diarrhea, abdominal cramps, and nausea. Probiotics can cause gas, bloating, and constipation, and some herbs and plant extracts can react negatively with pharmaceuticals.

When taking drugs and supplements to manage kidney health, it is critical to check with a healthcare expert. A healthcare professional can keep track of the medications and supplements you're taking, examine potential interactions, and change dosage and frequency as needed. Furthermore, people with kidney problems should exercise caution when taking supplements because their kidneys may not be able to digest them adequately.

In conclusion, drugs and supplements play an important role in renal health management, but it is critical to recognize the potential side effects and reactions that may arise. Regular check-ins with a healthcare practitioner can help people with kidney disease use drugs and supplements to support their kidney health in a safe manner.

Conclusion

Summary of key points about understanding medications and supplements for kidney health.

Understanding the function of drugs and supplements in renal health management is critical for people with chronic kidney disease (CKD) who want to enhance their overall health and well-being. Medications and vitamins can help to control symptoms, reduce the progression of kidney disease, and enhance overall health.

When contemplating drugs and supplements, working with a healthcare provider is vital since they can help evaluate what is appropriate for the individual's specific health needs. They can also keep track of and modify medications and dosages as necessary.

Angiotensin-converting enzyme inhibitors (ACE inhibitors), angiotensin receptor blockers (ARBs), diuretics, calcium channel blockers, and phosphorus binders are common drugs used to

Juicing for Kidney Health

treat renal disease. Supplements such as vitamin D and iron are also regularly used to improve kidney health.

Supplements that are thought to enhance kidney function include omega-3 fatty acids, magnesium, vitamin C, probiotics, and herbs and plant extracts. However, issues like dosage and frequency, potential interactions with other drugs and supplements, and adverse effects must all be considered.

Individuals with renal illness should frequently monitor their prescriptions and supplements, visit their healthcare providers on a regular basis, and be aware of any potential side effects or reactions.

To summarize, integrating drugs and supplements as part of a complete strategy for kidney health management is critical to helping improve health outcomes. It is critical to collaborate closely with a healthcare professional to decide what is appropriate for the individual's specific health needs and to assess and change as needed on a frequent basis.

The role of medications and supplements in a comprehensive approach to managing kidney disease.

Medications and vitamins are essential in the treatment of renal disease. They can help slow the progression of the disease and improve overall health when used correctly and in conjunction with other treatments and lifestyle modifications.

Kidney illness impairs a person's capacity to filter waste and excess fluids from the blood, which can result in a toxic accumulation in the body. Angiotensin-converting enzyme inhibitors (ACE inhibitors) and angiotensin receptor blockers (ARBs) are medications that can help manage blood pressure and protect the kidneys. Diuretics can also be used to eliminate excess fluid from the body, and calcium channel blockers and phosphorus binders can help balance these levels in the blood.

Supplements, in addition to drugs, can assist in promoting kidney health. Omega-3 fatty acids, magnesium, vitamin C, and probiotics have all been linked to improved kidney function. Herbs and plant extracts like ginger and turmeric may also be beneficial.

Juicing for Kidney Health

Individuals with renal illness should consult with their healthcare providers before selecting and utilizing drugs and supplements. Dosage and frequency, as well as any potential interactions with other medications, should be closely monitored. Check-ins with healthcare specialists on a regular basis can help ensure that the therapies and supplements being utilized are both successful and safe.

Incorporating drugs and supplements into a complete approach to kidney disease care, which may also include exercise, a balanced diet, and stress management, can help improve general health and decrease disease progression.

It's critical to remember that everyone's experience with kidney illness is different, and what works for one person might not work for another. Working with a healthcare practitioner to develop a personalized treatment plan is essential for determining the best combination of drugs and supplements to maintain kidney function.

Final thoughts on the importance of managing medications and supplements in supporting kidney health.

The function of drugs and supplements in renal health management is critical for people with chronic kidney disease (CKD), as they help to decrease disease progression and enhance overall health and quality of life. Medication and supplement management requires a complete approach that includes regular monitoring and check-ins with a healthcare provider.

Specific symptoms of kidney illness, such as high blood pressure, anemia, and bone disease, can be treated with medications and supplements, as well as improving overall health and well-being. Angiotensin-converting enzyme inhibitors (ACE inhibitors), angiotensin receptor blockers (ARBs), diuretics, calcium channel blockers, and phosphorus binders are common drugs used to treat renal disease. Vitamin D and iron supplements are also frequently used to treat dietary deficits.

Supplements like omega-3 fatty acids, magnesium, vitamin C, probiotics, and herbs and plant extracts are also frequently used to enhance kidney function. However, keep in mind that

Juicing for Kidney Health

supplements are not regulated by the FDA, and their efficacy and safety are not necessarily verified by scientific studies. As a result, it is critical to select supplements carefully and to check with a healthcare expert before beginning any new supplement program.

Incorporating drugs and supplements into a complete strategy for renal disease management necessitates thinking about dosage, frequency, and potential interactions with other medications. It is also critical to evaluate medications and supplements on a regular basis and to be mindful of side effects and potential responses.

Finally, controlling drugs and supplements is a vital part of maintaining kidney health. Individuals with CKD can benefit from regular consultation with a healthcare specialist and thorough consideration of all factors involved. Individuals with CKD can improve their health, delay the progression of the disease, and maintain a high quality of life by combining drugs, vitamins, and lifestyle adjustments.

Juicing for Kidney Health

CHAPTER 13

The Importance of Monitoring Kidney Function

Definition of Kidney Function

The kidneys are two bean-shaped organs on each side of the belly. They are in charge of filtering waste and other toxins from the blood and removing them from the body via urine. The kidneys also generate hormones that help regulate blood pressure, red blood cell formation, and calcium absorption for healthy bones. Furthermore, the kidneys are in charge of balancing the body's fluids and electrolytes.

All of the organs, including the kidneys, work together to keep the body in balance when it is healthy. The kidneys filter the blood, removing waste and other poisons. They also aid in the maintenance of fluid balance in the body by releasing hormones that regulate the quantity of water and salt in the body. The kidneys also create an enzyme called renin, which aids in blood pressure regulation.

The kidneys are also in charge of creating an active form of vitamin D, which aids in calcium absorption for healthy bones. As the kidneys filter the blood, they also create erythropoietin, a hormone that aids in the regulation of red blood cell synthesis.

The kidneys are constantly filtering blood and removing waste from the body. If the kidneys become damaged or diseased, they may be unable to adequately filter waste. This might result in the accumulation of waste products, which can cause major health issues. Regular examinations and tests can aid in the early detection and treatment of renal issues.

Overview of Kidney Function and its Importance

Kidney function is divided into three distinct processes: filtration, reabsorption, and secretion. The kidneys filter waste and surplus fluids from the blood into urine, which is ultimately excreted from the body. Important molecules, such as glucose, amino acids, and water, are also

Juicing for Kidney Health

reabsorbed by the kidneys and returned to the bloodstream for use by the organism. Finally, the kidneys secrete waste materials into the urine, such as urea.

The kidneys are also important in regulating blood pressure, generating red blood cells, and maintaining electrolyte balance in the body. They also create hormones that control calcium metabolism, red blood cell formation, and blood pressure.

One of the most important jobs of the kidneys is to maintain the body's electrolyte balance. Electrolytes such as sodium, potassium, and calcium are essential for numerous biological functions such as muscular contraction, fluid balance, and nerve signal transmission. The kidneys aid in the regulation of electrolyte levels in the blood by filtering out excess amounts and reabsorbing what the body requires.

It is crucial to maintain proper kidney function since the kidneys play an important role in general health and well-being. Chronic kidney disease (CKD) is a prevalent disorder in which the kidneys gradually lose function. If untreated, CKD can progress to renal failure, necessitating dialysis or a kidney transplant to sustain life.

High blood pressure, diabetes, a family history of renal disease, and age are all risk factors for developing CKD. Maintaining a healthy lifestyle, which includes eating a balanced diet, regulating blood pressure, and exercising on a regular basis, can help reduce the chance of developing CKD and retain kidney function.

Finally, the kidneys are vital organs that carry out a range of key duties in the body. Maintaining healthy kidney function is critical for general health and well-being, and taking efforts to reduce your risk of developing chronic renal disease can help you keep your kidney function for a lifetime.

Anatomy and Physiology of the Kidneys.

Structural Overview of the Kidneys.

The kidneys are complicated and highly specialized organs that are essential to the body's overall health and well-being. They are found in the lower back, on either side of the spine, and are protected by a layer of fat.

Juicing for Kidney Health

They are structurally separated into numerous parts, including the cortex, medulla, and pelvis. The cortex is the outer layer of the kidney and is responsible for the majority of waste products and excess fluid filtration from the blood. The medulla is the inner layer of the kidney and is in charge of urine production as well as fluid balance regulation in the body. The pelvis is a funnel-like structure that collects and carries urine from the kidney to the bladder.

The renal columns, renal pyramids, and renal papilla are among the components that comprise the cortex. The renal columns extend vertically through the cortex and contain the renal tubules, which are in charge of blood filtration and reabsorption. The renal pyramids are cone-shaped structures that serve as the foundation for the renal columns and house the renal papilla. The renal papilla is the location in the pelvis where urine produced by the kidneys is collected for excretion from the body.

The filtration process in the kidneys is aided by nephrons, which are the kidney's functional units. Each kidney includes around one million nephrons, which filter waste products and excess fluids from the blood. The glomerulus, a network of microscopic blood veins, is surrounded by the Bowman's capsule, which filters the blood. The glomerulus filters blood into the Bowman's capsule, where waste products and excess fluids are separated and collected in the renal tubules.

The renal tubules are in charge of reabsorbing vital nutrients back into the bloodstream, such as glucose, amino acids, and water. They also secrete waste materials into the urine, such as urea. The renal tubules are also in charge of maintaining the body's electrolyte balance, which includes sodium, potassium, and calcium.

In essence, the kidneys are complicated and highly specialized organs that play an important part in the body's overall health and well-being. Understanding the structural overview of the kidneys is vital for appreciating the intricate activities that occur within them, including filtration, reabsorption, and secretion, as well as their critical role in controlling the balance of substances in the body.

Juicing for Kidney Health

Mechanism of Kidney Function.

The mechanism of kidney function is a complicated and highly specialized process that is critical to the body's overall health and well-being. The kidneys filter waste materials and surplus fluids from the blood, regulate the balance of numerous substances, and conduct a variety of critical processes such as blood pressure regulation and red blood cell production.

The glomerulus, a network of microscopic blood vessels situated within the Bowman's capsule, is where the filtration process in the kidneys begins. The glomerulus filters blood into the Bowman's capsule, where waste products and excess fluids are separated. This filtered fluid, known as filtrate, is subsequently processed in the renal tubules and either reabsorbed into the bloodstream or removed from the body as urine.

The active movement of essential molecules such as glucose, amino acids, and water back into the bloodstream occurs during the reabsorption process in the kidneys. This is done by specialized cells in the renal tubules, which use ATP energy to pump the necessary chemicals back into the bloodstream.

The secretion process in the kidneys involves the removal of waste materials from the blood into the urine, such as urea. This is performed by specialized cells secreting waste materials into the renal tubules, where they are ultimately removed from the body in the urine.

The kidneys are also important in managing the balance of electrolytes in the body, such as sodium, potassium, and calcium. They accomplish this by removing excess levels of these compounds and reabsorbing what the body requires. The kidneys maintain this balance through a combination of filtration, reabsorption, and secretion mechanisms.

They also play a role in blood pressure regulation by producing hormones such as renin and erythropoietin. Renin controls blood pressure by managing the quantity of sodium and water in the body, whereas erythropoietin increases red blood cell synthesis in the bone marrow.

In summary, the mechanism of kidney function is a complicated and highly specialized process that is critical to the body's overall health and well-being. The kidneys filter waste materials and surplus fluids from the blood, regulate the balance of numerous substances, and conduct a variety of critical processes such as blood pressure regulation and red blood cell production.

Juicing for Kidney Health

Understanding the mechanism of kidney function is essential for appreciating the fundamental role the kidneys play in preserving health and well-being.

Importance of Monitoring Kidney Function.

Early Detection of Kidney Disease.

Early identification of renal illness is crucial for limiting disease progression and preserving kidney function. Kidney illness frequently has no symptoms in the early stages, and by the time symptoms show, the kidney damage may be permanent. Early detection and treatment can help decrease disease progression, avoid or postpone the onset of renal failure, and improve overall health outcomes.

Routine blood and urine testing, imaging examinations, and risk factor screening are all techniques for the early identification of kidney disease. The creatinine test, which detects the level of creatinine, a waste product, in the blood, is one of the most popular diagnostics for the early identification of renal disease. High creatinine levels may suggest that the kidneys are not working properly.

A urine test that analyzes the quantities of protein in the urine, such as albumin, is another common test for the early identification of kidney disease. Protein in the urine could mean that the kidneys aren't working properly and that waste products aren't being filtered effectively.

Ultrasound, CT scans, and MRI scans can also be used to detect kidney disease in its early stages. These tests can help detect changes in kidney size or shape, as well as the presence of tumors or other abnormal growths.

Another crucial part of early identification of renal disease is risk factor screening. High blood pressure, diabetes, and a family history of renal disease can all raise the chance of getting kidney disease. Regular screening for these risk factors can aid in the early detection of renal disease and timely treatment.

Aside from normal testing and screening, it is critical to get medical assistance if you have any symptoms of kidney disease, such as fatigue, lack of appetite, edema, or changes in urine output. Early therapy and lifestyle adjustments, such as limiting salt consumption, maintaining a healthy

Juicing for Kidney Health

weight, and controlling blood sugar levels, can help reduce the course of renal disease and preserve kidney function.

Early identification of kidney illness is crucial for limiting disease development and preserving renal function. Regular testing, imaging tests, and risk factor screening can help detect kidney disease in its early stages, and rapid treatment and lifestyle adjustments can help slow the illness's course and improve overall health outcomes. It is critical to get medical assistance if you have any concerns regarding your kidney function.

Evaluation of Kidney Function in Disease Management.

Evaluation of renal function is an important part of controlling and monitoring kidney illness. The kidneys filter waste materials and surplus fluids from the blood, regulate the balance of numerous substances, and conduct a variety of critical processes such as blood pressure regulation and red blood cell production. It is critical to appropriately diagnose and monitor kidney function in order to effectively manage renal disease.

Blood tests, urine tests, and imaging investigations are some of the methods used to assess kidney function. The creatinine test, for example, measures the level of creatinine, a waste product, in the blood. High creatinine levels may suggest that the kidneys are not working properly.

Urine testing can also tell you a lot about your kidney function. A urine test can detect protein levels in the urine, such as albumin. Protein in the urine could mean that the kidneys aren't working properly and that waste products aren't being filtered effectively.

Ultrasounds, CT scans, and MRI scans can also provide useful information on kidney function. These tests can help detect changes in kidney size or shape, as well as the presence of tumors or other abnormal growths.

In addition to these tests, it is critical to monitor other factors that can affect kidney function, such as blood pressure, blood sugar levels, and electrolyte levels. Regular monitoring of these variables can aid in the detection of abnormalities in kidney function and quick therapy.

Juicing for Kidney Health

Treatment for kidney disease varies according to its severity and underlying cause. Kidney disease can be controlled early on with lifestyle adjustments such as limiting salt intake, maintaining a healthy weight, and regulating blood sugar levels. Treatment for advanced kidney disease may include medication, dialysis, or kidney transplantation.

Finally, assessing kidney function is a crucial part of managing renal disease and tracking its progression. Regular testing, monitoring of risk factors, and quick treatment can all help delay disease progression and preserve kidney function. It is critical to get medical assistance if you have any concerns regarding your kidney function. Your healthcare professional can assist you in assessing your kidney function and determining the best course of treatment for your specific needs.

Monitoring of Kidney Function in Chronic Kidney Disease.

Monitoring kidney function is crucial for controlling and preventing the progression of chronic kidney disease (CKD). CKD is a chronic disorder that inhibits the kidneys' capacity to function normally. CKD can progress to renal failure over time, necessitating dialysis or kidney transplantation to preserve life. Regular monitoring of kidney function can aid in the detection of disease changes and quick therapy.

Blood tests, urine tests, and imaging investigations are some of the modalities used to monitor kidney function in people with CKD. The creatinine test, for example, measures the level of creatinine, a waste product, in the blood. High creatinine levels may suggest that the kidneys are not working properly.

Urine testing can also tell you a lot about your kidney function. A urine test can detect protein levels in the urine, such as albumin. Protein in the urine could mean that the kidneys aren't working properly and that waste products aren't being filtered effectively.

Ultrasounds, CT scans, and MRI scans can also provide useful information on kidney function. These tests can help detect changes in kidney size or shape, as well as the presence of tumors or other abnormal growths.

Juicing for Kidney Health

In addition to these tests, it is critical to monitor other factors that can affect kidney function, such as blood pressure, blood sugar levels, and electrolyte levels. Regular monitoring of these variables can aid in the detection of abnormalities in kidney function and quick therapy.

Treatment for CKD varies based on the severity of the disease and the underlying cause. CKD can be controlled by lifestyle changes such as limiting salt intake, maintaining a healthy weight, and regulating blood sugar levels in its early stages. Treatment for advanced CKD may include medication, dialysis, or kidney transplantation.

If you have CKD, you should see your doctor on a regular basis for monitoring and evaluation of your kidney function. Your healthcare professional can assist you in monitoring your kidney function, tracking disease progression, and determining the best course of treatment for your specific needs. Regular monitoring of renal function is essential for preventing disease development and preserving kidney function.

Finally, monitoring kidney function is an important part of controlling and preventing the progression of chronic kidney disease (CKD). Regular testing, monitoring of risk factors, and quick treatment can all help delay disease progression and preserve kidney function. If you have CKD, you should see your doctor on a regular basis for monitoring and evaluation of your kidney function.

Importance of Kidney Function Monitoring in Drug Therapy

Kidney function testing is essential in medication therapy since the kidneys are responsible for removing waste products and excess fluids from the body. The kidneys process and eliminate many drugs, and changes in renal function can alter the elimination and effectiveness of many medications. As a result, monitoring kidney function is crucial in ensuring that individuals receive the proper dose of medication and that the medication is not harming the kidneys.

Drugs can have a variety of effects on kidney function. Some medicines can cause direct kidney damage, while others might increase the stress on the kidneys, resulting in reduced function. Changes in kidney function can, in some situations, modify the pharmacokinetics of medications, affecting their clearance rate and effectiveness.

Juicing for Kidney Health

It is critical to evaluate renal function before and during medication therapy to minimize these potential problems. This can assist in detecting changes in renal function that may alter drug elimination and effectiveness, allowing necessary adjustments to the amount or type of medication to be made.

Blood tests, urine tests, and imaging examinations are all approaches for assessing kidney function. The creatinine test, for example, measures the level of creatinine, a waste product, in the blood. High creatinine levels may suggest that the kidneys are not working properly.

Urine testing can also tell you a lot about your kidney function. A urine test can detect protein levels in the urine, such as albumin. Protein in the urine could mean that the kidneys aren't working properly and that waste products aren't being filtered effectively.

Ultrasounds, CT scans, and MRI scans can also provide useful information on kidney function. These tests can help detect changes in kidney size or shape, as well as the presence of tumors or other abnormal growths.

Monitoring kidney function is critical in medication therapy since changes in renal function can alter drug removal and effectiveness. Regular testing and monitoring of kidney function can help ensure that people are getting the right dose of medication and that the medication isn't harming their kidneys. If you are taking medication, it is critical that you see your doctor on a frequent basis for monitoring and evaluation of your kidney function. Your doctor can assist you in monitoring your kidney function and ensuring that the medicine you are taking is safe and effective.

Methods of Monitoring Kidney Function.

Laboratory Tests.

Laboratory tests are critical in monitoring kidney function. These tests can provide vital information about kidney health and aid in the detection of early indicators of kidney illness or dysfunction.

Some of the most regularly used laboratory tests for assessing kidney function are as follows:

Juicing for Kidney Health

Creatinine test: This test determines the amount of creatinine in the blood. Creatinine is a waste product excreted by the kidneys that is created by the muscles. Creatinine levels in the blood may be elevated if the kidneys are not functioning normally.

The blood urea nitrogen (BUN) test determines the amount of urea nitrogen in the blood. Urea nitrogen is a waste product created by the body when protein is broken down. High urea nitrogen levels in the blood may suggest that the kidneys are not working properly.

Glomerular filtration rate (GFR) test: The GFR test determines how quickly the kidneys filter blood. This test gives an accurate assessment of overall kidney function. A low GFR could indicate that the kidneys aren't working properly.

Urine testing can provide valuable information on kidney function. A urine test can detect protein levels in the urine, such as albumin. Protein in the urine could mean that the kidneys aren't working properly and that waste products aren't being filtered effectively.

Electrolyte testing: Electrolyte tests evaluate the amounts of minerals in the blood, such as sodium, potassium, and calcium. In renal disease, electrolyte imbalances can arise, and these tests can help detect and monitor these abnormalities.

Urinalysis: Urinalysis is a comprehensive test that can reveal vital information about the kidney's health. The presence of protein, blood, and other waste products in the urine can be detected by the test, which may suggest kidney illness or dysfunction.

It is crucial to emphasize that laboratory testing is only one component of assessing kidney function. Other tests, such as imaging investigations and physical examinations, may be required to obtain an accurate picture of kidney function.

Laboratory testing is crucial for monitoring kidney function. Regular testing can aid in the early detection of kidney illness or dysfunction, allowing for rapid treatment and management. If you have a history of renal disease or are at risk for kidney disease, you should talk to your doctor about the importance of regular kidney function tests. Based on your unique needs and medical history, your healthcare practitioner can assist you in determining the optimal testing schedule for you.

Juicing for Kidney Health

Imaging tests are an important technique for evaluating kidney function and can provide crucial information about kidney health. These tests can detect changes in the kidney's structure and size, as well as abnormalities in blood flow to the kidneys.

Some of the most often utilized imaging diagnostics for assessing kidney function are as follows:

Ultrasound is a non-invasive imaging test that creates images of the kidneys using high-frequency sound waves. Ultrasound can be used to assess kidney size and shape, as well as identify changes in blood flow to the kidneys.

A CT scan is a non-invasive imaging technique that employs X-rays and computer processing to produce detailed images of the kidneys. CT scans can provide extensive information about the size and shape of the kidneys, as well as aid in the detection of abnormalities in blood flow to the kidneys.

Magnetic resonance imaging (MRI): MRI is a non-invasive imaging test that creates detailed images of the kidneys using a strong magnetic field, radio waves, and computer processing. MRI can provide detailed information on the kidney's anatomy and function, as well as measure blood flow to the kidneys.

Angiography: An invasive imaging technique that employs X-rays and a contrast dye to provide detailed images of the blood arteries in the kidneys. Angiography can be used to assess blood flow to the kidneys and to detect blockages or constriction of the kidney's blood arteries.

Renal scintigraphy is a non-invasive imaging procedure that creates images of blood flow to the kidneys using a small amount of radioactive material and a particular camera. Renal scintigraphy is a technique for evaluating blood flow to the kidneys and detecting changes in blood flow to the kidneys.

Juicing for Kidney Health

It is crucial to emphasize that imaging tests are only one component of assessing renal function. Other diagnostics, such as laboratory tests and physical examinations, may be required to obtain an accurate picture of kidney function.

In conclusion, imaging examinations are critical in evaluating kidney function. Regular imaging studies can detect changes in kidney size and structure, as well as changes in blood flow to the kidneys. If you have a history of renal disease or are at risk for kidney disease, you should talk to your doctor about the importance of regular kidney function tests. Based on your unique needs and medical history, your healthcare practitioner can assist you in determining the appropriate imaging test schedule for you.

Kidney Biopsy.

A kidney biopsy is a procedure used to examine and diagnose kidney diseases. It entails obtaining a sample of kidney tissue and studying it under a microscope for evidence of injury or disease. A kidney biopsy can provide vital information about the kidney's health and aid in the identification and monitoring of disorders such as renal disease or kidney failure.

A doctor or expert performs the procedure in a hospital or clinic. It is usually performed under local anesthesia, which means that the patient is awake but the area around the biopsy site is numbed. To obtain a small sample of tissue, a thin, hollow needle is passed through the skin and into the kidney. The sample is subsequently delivered to a laboratory for analysis and testing.

A kidney biopsy can aid in the diagnosis and monitoring of a variety of illnesses, including:

• Kidney calcifications

• Kidney inflammation or infection

• Kidney disease

• Glomerulonephritis (a type of kidney disease) is a type of kidney disease.

• Lupus Nephropathy (an autoimmune condition that affects the kidneys)

• Kidney vascular disorders

Juicing for Kidney Health

• Rejection of a kidney transplant

• Kidney illness that is chronic

• Kidney injury, acute

A kidney biopsy can provide vital information about the kidney's health and help make decisions about the best course of treatment for the patient. It can also be used to track changes in the kidney over time in order to ensure that any treatment is effective and to identify any potential problems.

Kidney biopsies are generally risk-free procedures with a low risk of significant consequences. However, the operation may include some dangers, such as bleeding, infection, and pain. Before the surgery, your doctor will go over any potential risks and adverse effects with you.

To summarize, a kidney biopsy is an effective and dependable means of assessing kidney function. It can provide crucial information about the kidney's health and assist in making decisions about the best course of treatment for the patient. It's a rather safe technique with a low chance of major consequences.

Assessment of Kidney Function through Clinical Signs and Symptoms.

The evaluation of kidney function is an important part of diagnosing and monitoring an individual's health. The kidneys filter waste and surplus fluids from the body, regulate blood pressure, and produce hormones that govern red blood cell development and bone health. As a result, any disturbance in kidney function can have serious consequences for an individual's overall health.

Clinical signs and symptoms are a valuable tool in determining kidney function. These signs and symptoms can help determine the extent and kind of kidney damage, as well as aid in the diagnosis of underlying disorders that may be interfering with renal function.

Changes in urine production are one of the most common clinical indicators of renal failure. Oliguria, or decreased urine output, can be an indication of impaired kidney function and may indicate the existence of acute renal injury or chronic kidney disease. An increase in urine

Juicing for Kidney Health

output, or polyuria, on the other hand, may suggest a problem with the body's maintenance of fluid balance, which can also compromise kidney function.

Proteinuria, or the presence of too much protein in the urine, is another symptom of renal disease. The kidneys filter waste items from the blood, and an excess of protein in the urine can suggest that the kidneys are not working properly. This can be an indication of a variety of underlying diseases, such as glomerulonephritis, diabetes, or hypertension.

Another typical indication of renal disease is edema, or swelling. This can happen when the kidneys are unable to manage fluid balance in the body adequately, resulting in excess fluid accumulation in the tissues. Edema can develop in a variety of locations throughout the body, including the legs, ankles, and face.

Another typical indication of renal disease is high blood pressure, sometimes known as hypertension. Hypertension can be caused by a variety of factors, including waste product accumulation in the blood and the synthesis of hormones that regulate blood pressure. Hypertension in people with renal impairment can be an indication of worsening kidney function and may indicate the need for more aggressive treatment.

Back pain, particularly in the lumbar region, might potentially indicate kidney failure. This pain can be caused by a number of underlying disorders, including infections, tumors, and kidney stones.

Kidney impairment can also cause nausea and vomiting, exhaustion, and a loss of appetite. These symptoms can occur as a result of waste product accumulation in the blood, which can cause feelings of malaise and lower energy levels.

Finally, clinical indications and symptoms are important in determining renal function. Changes in urine output, proteinuria, edema, hypertension, back pain, nausea and vomiting, exhaustion, and decreased appetite are all symptoms of renal failure and may indicate the existence of other disorders affecting kidney function. If you are having any of these symptoms, it is critical that you consult with your doctor to discover the cause and obtain the right treatment.

Juicing for Kidney Health

Factors that Affect Kidney Function

Age and Genetics

Two key factors that can alter kidney function are age and heredity. Kidneys filter waste and extra fluid from the body, so when these organs aren't working properly, it can lead to a number of health issues.

The kidneys are made up of many nephrons, which are microscopic filters that help separate waste and excess fluid from the blood. The number of nephrons in our kidneys diminishes as we age, resulting in a decrease in filtering capability. This is why, in order to help their kidneys perform as efficiently as possible, older persons should drink enough fluids and maintain a balanced diet.

In addition to age, genetics can influence how well the kidneys work. Certain hereditary diseases, such as polycystic kidney disease, can make the kidneys less effective at filtering waste, resulting in a toxic accumulation in the body. People with a family history of renal disease should be extremely cautious, and they should consult their doctor about strategies to keep their kidneys healthy.

Aside from age and genetics, lifestyle variables might influence how well the kidneys work. Obese people, smokers, and people with one of the illnesses associated with chronic kidney disease (such as diabetes or hypertension) are at a higher risk of developing renal difficulties. A nutritious diet, frequent exercise, and maintaining a healthy weight can all help lower the risk of kidney diseases.

Overall, age and genetics can impact kidney function, but adopting a healthy lifestyle can help to prevent or slow the progression of kidney disease. People who are at risk should consult with their doctor about measures to keep their kidneys as healthy and functional as possible.

Lifestyle and Environmental Factors

A range of lifestyle and environmental factors influence kidney function. The kidneys filter waste and fluid from the body, and their capacity to do so might be hampered by certain habits

Juicing for Kidney Health

and exposures. Knowing which lifestyle and environmental factors can affect kidney function can help people make informed health and well-being decisions.

Diet, in particular, can have a significant impact on kidney health. A well-balanced diet rich in fruits, vegetables, and whole grains aids in the normal functioning of the kidneys. Consuming too much salt or processed meat, on the other hand, can place a burden on the kidneys, potentially leading to a variety of health concerns. Furthermore, excessive alcohol consumption can harm the kidneys since alcohol is a diuretic, which means it increases the amount of urine generated.

Exercise is also helpful for keeping your kidneys healthy. Regular physical exercise aids the body's elimination of toxins, reducing the stress on the kidneys. Exercise can also help lower blood pressure, which is another issue that might impact kidney function.

Environmental factors might also have an adverse effect on renal function. Certain chemicals, such as those contained in solvents and insecticides, can cause kidney injury. Furthermore, both air pollution and heavy metal exposure might damage kidney function.

Many drugs and medical conditions might be harmful to the kidneys. Nonsteroidal anti-inflammatory medicines, such as ibuprofen, can cause kidney damage if taken in significant amounts. Diabetes, high blood pressure, and lupus, among other disorders, can all compromise kidney function.

Finally, it is important to understand how lifestyle and environmental factors influence kidney function. Eating a balanced diet, exercising regularly, and avoiding certain chemicals and pollutants can all help to keep the kidneys in good working order. Furthermore, people should be aware of any medications they are taking as well as any medical issues they may have, as these can all have an impact on kidney function.

Medical Conditions

Medical disorders can have a significant impact on kidney function. Diabetes, hypertension, and autoimmune illnesses can all result in chronic kidney disease (CKD) and kidney failure.

Juicing for Kidney Health

Diabetes, in particular, is the primary cause of CKD in the United States and other industrialized countries, with an estimated one-third of diabetics developing some type of CKD.

High blood pressure can also impair renal function significantly. Hypertension (high blood pressure) is a major risk factor for CKD and can cause a number of kidney-related issues, such as proteinuria (excess protein in the urine), glomerulonephritis (inflammation of the glomeruli, the microscopic filtering units of the kidney), and an increased risk of kidney stones.

Lupus and IgA nephropathy are two autoimmune disorders that can cause kidney damage. Lupus is an autoimmune condition in which the immune system targets the body's own cells, particularly kidney cells. IgA nephropathy is an autoimmune condition that causes the body to create antibodies that attack the filtering units of the kidneys, causing inflammation and damage.

Medication, environmental pollutants, and some types of infections, such as those caused by the bacteria Streptococcus, can also cause kidney impairment. Toxins in the environment, such as lead, mercury, cadmium, and arsenic, can also impair kidney function, leading to chronic renal disease.

Finally, kidney failure can be caused by a number of other disorders, including inherited diseases like polycystic kidney disease and genetic abnormalities like Alport syndrome. These disorders can cause irreparable kidney damage and, in certain situations, can be fatal.

Medical disorders can have a significant impact on kidney function, and it is critical for people to understand their risk of developing chronic renal disease or kidney failure. If you have any of the illnesses listed above, you should be aware of the potential consequences for your kidneys and keep an eye on their health.

Medications and Drugs.

Drugs and medications can have a significant impact on kidney function. Certain drugs, in some cases, can increase the risk of kidney damage or failure. Medication can also be used to treat a range of renal diseases in other circumstances. To make informed treatment decisions, it is critical to understand how medications and substances can alter renal function. To begin, it is critical to realize that the kidneys are in charge of filtering waste and excess fluid from the body.

Juicing for Kidney Health

They also help to regulate blood pressure and release hormones. Medication can have an effect on how the kidneys function, either positively or adversely. Certain medications, such as nonsteroidal anti-inflammatory drugs (NSAIDs) and antibiotics, have been linked to an increased risk of renal issues in some people. NSAIDs can raise the risk of renal injury, whereas antibiotics can cause kidney function to decline.

It is vital to discuss any medications you are taking with your doctor, as well as the dangers associated with them. Medication can be used to address renal disorders in some circumstances. Diuretic medicines, for example, can be used to minimize edema caused by excess fluid in the body. These drugs function by boosting urine production, which aids in the removal of excess fluid. Anemia, a common sign of kidney illness, can be treated with other drugs such as erythropoietin. Before taking any medications or supplements that may impact your kidneys, consult with your doctor.

Your doctor can advise you on the best way to manage your kidney health, including any necessary lifestyle adjustments. They can also help you analyze the hazards of any medications or supplements you are thinking about using. Drugs and medications can have a significant impact on renal function. It is critical to understand how these medications can impact the kidneys and to discuss any medications or supplements you are contemplating taking with your doctor. Even with medications or supplements, it is possible to maintain healthy kidney function with careful management.

Summary of Key Points.

The significance of monitoring kidney function cannot be overemphasized because the kidneys play an important part in general health and well-being. They are in charge of removing waste and excess fluid from the blood, balancing electrolytes, creating hormones that control red blood cell production and blood pressure, and much more. When kidney function begins to diminish, it can lead to a variety of health issues, making it critical to monitor renal function on a frequent basis.

Here are some important aspects to consider when monitoring kidney function:

Juicing for Kidney Health

1. Be aware of your risk factors: Certain variables, such as high blood pressure, diabetes, a family history of kidney disease, and advancing age, increase the chance of developing kidney disease. If you have any of these risk factors, you should get your kidney function evaluated on a regular basis.

2. Regular testing: A creatinine blood test and a glomerular filtration rate (GFR) test are the most common tests used to assess kidney function. Regular testing can aid in the early detection of issues, when they are easier to cure.

3. Be on the lookout for signs and symptoms: Although kidney disease frequently proceeds silently, there are some indications to be aware of, such as weariness, swelling in the legs and ankles, decreased urine production, and changes in the frequency or appearance of urine. If you encounter any of these symptoms, you should seek medical assistance right away.

Sustaining a healthy lifestyle is vital for maintaining excellent kidney function. Maintaining a healthy weight, eating a balanced diet, and exercising regularly are all part of it. Controlling any underlying health issues, such as high blood pressure and diabetes, is particularly critical, as these can contribute to kidney damage.

5.Medications and treatments: Because certain medications and treatments can harm the kidneys, it's critical to discuss any medications or treatments you're using with your doctor.They can help you assess if they are hurting your kidney function and, if so, advise alternate solutions.

Finally, monitoring kidney function is an important part of maintaining overall health and well-being. You can help ensure that your kidneys continue to work well by identifying your risk factors, getting frequent testing, checking for signs and symptoms, maintaining a healthy lifestyle, and being careful of any drugs or treatments you are taking. Early detection and treatment of renal disorders can considerably increase management success and avoid kidney disease development. Make an appointment with your healthcare professional to discuss the best monitoring plan for you.

Juicing for Kidney Health

Juicing for Kidney Health

CHAPTER 14

14

Overview of the importance of maintaining kidney health.

It is impossible to overestimate the significance of sustaining renal health. Our kidneys are critical organs that filter waste and surplus fluids from our bloodstream, regulate electrolyte balance, produce hormones that govern red blood cell development, control blood pressure, and aid in bone health. Unfortunately, kidney disease is a frequent and significant health problem, with millions of people suffering from renal failure each year throughout the world. Maintaining kidney health is critical for preventing renal disease and ensuring that the kidneys continue to function correctly.

Sustaining a healthy lifestyle is one of the most critical measures for maintaining kidney health. This involves eating a balanced, low-salt diet, not smoking, and engaging in frequent physical activity. It is also critical to monitor and manage illnesses like high blood pressure and diabetes, which can raise the risk of renal disease. Furthermore, staying hydrated and drinking plenty of water are vital for flushing out waste and preventing the buildup of toxic compounds in the kidneys.

Regular visits to a healthcare provider are also essential for preserving kidney health. Regular blood and urine tests to monitor kidney function, as well as screenings for illnesses that can raise the risk of renal disease, such as high blood pressure, diabetes, and heart disease, are part of this. In some circumstances, imaging tests such as an ultrasound, CT scan, or MRI may be required to provide a better understanding of the kidneys' condition.

Early detection and treatment of renal illness are critical for preventing its progression and maintaining kidney function. Medication to lower blood pressure and manage symptoms, lifestyle modifications such as eating a balanced diet, and, in severe situations, dialysis or a kidney transplant are common therapies for kidney disease.

Juicing for Kidney Health

In addition to individual efforts, greater public awareness and investment in kidney health are required. This involves expanding access to early detection and treatment, offering education and resources to individuals with kidney disease, and investing in research to create novel kidney disease treatments and solutions.

In conclusion, preserving kidney health is critical for ensuring that these key organs continue to operate normally and preventing the development of kidney disease. Healthy lifestyle choices, regular check-ups with a healthcare practitioner, early identification and treatment of kidney disease, and improved public knowledge and investment in kidney health can all help to preserve kidney function and prevent renal disease development.

The role of juicing in supporting kidney health.

Juicing has grown in popularity as a technique to improve general health and wellness, and its benefits for kidney health are worth investigating. The kidneys are essential organs that filter waste and surplus fluids from our bloodstream, regulate electrolyte balance, produce hormones that regulate red blood cell development, and regulate blood pressure. Kidney function is critical for general health and well-being.

It offers the body a plethora of vitamins, minerals, and antioxidants, which is one of its many advantages. Many of these nutrients, such as vitamins C and E, as well as minerals like potassium, magnesium, and calcium, are needed for kidney health. Antioxidants, such as those found in dark, leafy greens, can also help protect the kidneys from oxidative stress damage.

It also gives the body an abundance of fluids, which is vital for kidney function. To efficiently filter waste and surplus fluids from the bloodstream, the kidneys require an appropriate amount of fluid. Drinking fresh juice can help increase fluid intake and hydration, which can improve kidney function.

In addition to important vitamins, minerals, and hydration, certain varieties of juice can improve kidney health by lowering inflammation and the risk of chronic kidney disease. Juices prepared from beets, cranberries, and pomegranates, for example, include chemicals that have been demonstrated to improve kidney health. Nitrates in beets have been demonstrated to lower blood pressure and enhance blood flow to the kidneys, whereas cranberries have been shown to

Juicing for Kidney Health

minimize the incidence of urinary tract infections, which can cause kidney damage over time. Pomegranates contain antioxidants that can help protect the kidneys from the effects of oxidative stress.

While juicing can be a beneficial supplement to a healthy diet, it should not be relied on as the primary source of nutrients. Juice is frequently lacking in protein, an important component for kidney function, and high in sugar. It is also critical to check the source of the juice, as certain commercial juices may have additional sugar or artificial sweeteners, both of which can be damaging to the kidneys.

In summary, juicing can benefit kidney health by providing the body with vital vitamins, minerals, fluids, and antioxidants. However, it should not be relied on as the sole source of nutrients, and the source of the juice as well as the overall balance of the diet should be considered. Regular check-ups with a healthcare professional, as well as a healthy lifestyle that includes a balanced diet, exercise, and stress management, are all critical for preserving kidney health and preventing the progression of renal disease.

Staying Motivated

Setting achievable goals.

It can be difficult to stay motivated and dedicated to adopting changes to support kidney health, especially when it comes to incorporating new habits like juicing. Setting attainable goals will help you stay on track and give you a sense of accomplishment along the way.

Being realistic about what you can really achieve is one of the first steps in defining feasible goals. It is critical to begin modestly and progressively increase the difficulty of your goals as you gain comfort and confidence in your talents. If your objective is to introduce more juicing into your diet, for example, you may begin by introducing one serving of juice into your daily routine and progressively increase the frequency and variety of juices as you become more comfortable.

Juicing for Kidney Health

Setting defined and quantifiable goals is also essential. Set a precise objective, such as "I will drink one serving of juice every day for the next week," rather than simply saying you want to drink more juice. This is a particular, quantifiable aim that can be easily tracked and evaluated.

Making a plan for how you will attain your goals is another important component of defining feasible goals. Setting aside specific hours each day for juicing, making a shopping list of ingredients, or finding recipes that you enjoy are all examples of this. You will be more likely to stay motivated and on track if you have a clear plan in place.

In addition to defining attainable goals, it is critical to stay motivated and dedicated to accomplishing them. Finding a support system, such as a friend or family member who is interested in juicing and kidney health, or joining a support group or community where you can share your experiences and receive encouragement and support, may be necessary.

Remember to reward yourself along the way. This might help you maintain motivation by reinforcing favorable habits. Small and easy rewards, such as treating yourself to a special dinner or engaging in a cherished hobby, will suffice.

Finally, creating attainable goals is critical to keeping motivated and committed to improving kidney health through juicing. Setting clear, quantifiable goals, establishing a plan for how you will reach your goals, finding a support system, and rewarding yourself along the way will help you stay motivated and on track. Be patient and nice to yourself, because transformation takes time and work. Celebrate your victories and gains along the way and keep working toward greater kidney health.

Tracking progress and celebrating successes.

Tracking progress and appreciating accomplishments are critical components of being motivated and committed to achieving kidney health through juicing. Monitoring progress can help to create a sense of success as well as a greater knowledge of what is working and what needs to be tweaked in order to meet your objectives. Celebrating little victories can provide motivation and reinforce desirable habits.

Juicing for Kidney Health

Keeping a journal is one way to keep track of your development. This can involve keeping track of the type and frequency with which you consume juice, as well as any changes in your overall health and well-being. This data can be utilized to spot patterns and make necessary changes to your juicing regimen.

Monitoring your physical health is another approach to tracking your development. This may entail keeping track of your blood pressure, weight, and other pertinent kidney health indicators. Working with a healthcare physician to track your progress and make any required changes is a crucial part of achieving renal health.

Celebrating accomplishments, no matter how minor, is a crucial part of remaining motivated. Recognizing and acknowledging modest steps toward your goals can help keep you motivated and committed to achieving kidney health through juicing. Setting up a reward system, such as treating yourself to a special meal or engaging in a favorite hobby after achieving a goal, or simply taking the time to recognize and celebrate your triumphs with friends and family, can help.

It is also critical to remember that growth is not always linear and that setbacks may occur along the way. During these times, it is critical to be patient and kind to yourself, focusing on what you have learned and what you can do differently in the future.

Keeping track of progress and celebrating victories are critical components of remaining motivated and committed to improving kidney health with juicing. You will be more likely to stay motivated and on track to achieve your goals if you keep a journal, check your physical health, and celebrate your victories.

Remember to be patient and nice to yourself, as well as to appreciate your accomplishments and progress along the way. It can be difficult to stay motivated and dedicated to adopting changes to support kidney health, especially when it comes to incorporating new habits like juicing. Setting attainable goals will help you stay on track and give you a sense of accomplishment along the way.

While juicing can be a beneficial supplement to a healthy diet, it should not be relied on as the primary source of nutrients. Juice is frequently lacking in protein, an important component for kidney function, and high in sugar. It is also critical to check the source of the juice, as certain

Juicing for Kidney Health

commercial juices may have additional sugar or artificial sweeteners, both of which can be damaging to the kidneys.

In summary, juicing can benefit kidney health by providing the body with vital vitamins, minerals, fluids, and antioxidants. However, it should not be relied on as the sole source of nutrients, and the source of the juice as well as the overall balance of the diet should be considered. Regular check-ups with a healthcare professional, as well as a healthy lifestyle that includes a balanced diet, exercise, and stress management, are all critical for preserving kidney health and preventing the progression of renal disease.

Surrounding oneself with positive support.

Surrounding oneself with good support is essential for staying motivated and dedicated to kidney health through juicing. Having a supportive network of friends, family, and healthcare providers can help you achieve your goals by providing encouragement, motivation, and accountability.

Involving friends and family in your journey to better kidney health is one method to create a support network. This could include telling them about your aims and experiences, or even inviting them to join you in implementing juicing into your daily routine. Having someone with whom you can share your experiences and keep you accountable can be a strong motivation.

It is also crucial to work with a healthcare physician who is supportive of your goals and educated about the function of juicing in promoting kidney health. Your healthcare practitioner can help you make changes to your food and lifestyle, as well as monitor your progress and make any required adjustments along the way.

Joining a kidney health or juicing support group or community can provide a supportive network. This can be a terrific opportunity to connect with others who are going through similar experiences and to receive encouragement and support from others who are on the same journey.

Finally, it is critical to surround yourself with positive self-talk and thinking. This could include confronting negative ideas and replacing them with positive affirmations, as well as searching out activities and experiences that offer you joy and happiness.

Juicing for Kidney Health

In summary, surrounding oneself with good support is critical to remaining motivated and devoted to improving kidney health through juicing. You will be more likely to stay motivated and on track to achieve your goals if you involve friends and family, work with a supportive healthcare professional, join a support group, and focus on positive self-talk and a positive mindset. Remember to seek out help and to appreciate your accomplishments along the road.

Finding inspiration and encouragement through community resources.

Getting inspiration and support from community resources can be a tremendous incentive for staying motivated and committed to improving kidney health through juicing. There are numerous tools available to help you achieve your goals by providing inspiration, guidance, and support.

Online communities and forums dedicated to kidney health and juicing are one such resource. These groups can help people connect with others who are going through similar things, share experiences and suggestions, and provide encouragement and support. This can be a terrific way to get inspired and motivated while also learning about new recipes and juicing processes.

Local activities and workshops on kidney health and juicing are another option. These events can provide opportunities to interact with others on a similar journey, hear from professionals in the industry, and be inspired and encouraged.

Reading books and articles about juicing and kidney health can also provide a lot of inspiration and motivation. This can help you understand the function of juicing in kidney health and provide practical advice and techniques for implementing juicing into your daily practice.

Finally, interacting with kidney health specialists and organizations can provide further resources and assistance. These organizations may provide instructional materials, support groups, and other tools to assist you in remaining motivated and on track toward your objectives.

Finally, seeking inspiration and support through community resources is an essential part of being motivated and committed to improving kidney health through juicing. You will be more likely to stay motivated and on track towards your goals if you participate in online groups, attend local events and seminars, read relevant materials, and interact with healthcare practitioners and organizations. Remember to seek out resources and assistance, as well as to celebrate your accomplishments and progress along the way.

Tips for Successful Juicing.

Choosing the right juicer.

Choosing the correct juicer is critical for those who want to incorporate juicing into their daily practice to improve kidney health. With so many options available, it might be difficult to select the best juicer for your needs. However, by taking a few essential criteria into account, you can pick the best juicer for you and set yourself up for success.

1.Juicer Type: Different types of juicers are available, including centrifugal juicers, masticating juicers, and twin gear juicers. Each type of juicer has its own set of advantages and disadvantages, so it is critical to choose the juicer that will best match your needs. Centrifugal juicers are an excellent choice for folks who are new to juicing and want a low-cost, easy-to-use solution. Masticating juicers are suitable for people who want the highest-quality juice and are willing to invest in a more expensive and advanced juicer, while dual-gear juicers are ideal for those who want the highest-quality juice and are willing to invest in a more expensive and advanced juicer.

2. Capacity: Another key factor to consider is the juicer's capacity. If you intend to juice for more than one person, buy a juicer with a higher capacity. A smaller capacity juicer, on the other hand, may be more appropriate if you are only juicing for yourself or one or two people.

3. Ease of Use and Cleaning: Because juicing can become a regular ritual, it is critical to select a juicer that is simple to use and clean. Look for a juicer with basic controls that can be quickly and easily removed and cleaned.

4. Price: The cost of a juicer is also an important factor to consider. While you may be tempted to buy the cheapest juicer available, keep in mind that you typically get what you pay for. A more expensive juicer may produce higher-quality juice and last longer, so consider the long-term cost of ownership when selecting a juicer.

Juicing for Kidney Health

5. Warranties: Finally, it is critical to analyze the manufacturer's warranty. A juicer with a longer warranty duration might provide peace of mind and may show that the manufacturer is confident in their product's quality.

In conclusion, selecting the correct juicer is critical for people wishing to incorporate juicing into their daily practice to support kidney health. You may pick the best juicer for you by taking into account criteria such as the type of juicer, capacity, simplicity of use and cleaning, pricing, and warranty.

Selecting the right ingredients.

The items you choose will have a direct impact on the quality of the juice and its benefits for your kidney health; therefore, choosing the appropriate ingredients is a vital element of successful juicing. To get the most out of your juicing regimen, use components that are both healthful and tasty.

1. Fruits and Veggies: When choosing fruits and vegetables for your juice, consider a variety of hues to guarantee you get a diversity of nutrients. Leafy greens, for example, like kale, spinach, and lettuce, are high in vitamins and minerals, whereas red and yellow fruits and vegetables, like bell peppers, carrots, and tomatoes, are high in antioxidants.

Berries, such as strawberries, blueberries, and blackberries, are strong in antioxidants and make an excellent addition to any juice mix. They're also low in sugar, making them a good choice for people who have kidney difficulties and need to limit their sugar intake.

3. Herbs and spices: Spices and herbs like ginger, turmeric, and mint can add taste and nutrition to your juice. They can also aid in reducing inflammation, which is essential for kidney function.

4. Protein: A source of protein, such as almond milk, Greek yogurt, or protein powder, can be added to your juice to make it a complete meal. This will help to keep you full and satisfied while also balancing the juice's sugar content.

5. Sweeteners: If you prefer, you can add a natural sweetener to your juice, such as stevia or honey. However, it is crucial to remember that too much sugar can be damaging to the kidneys, so restrict the quantity of sweetness you use.

Juicing for Kidney Health

6. Avoiding Certain Substances: Some ingredients should be avoided when juicing since they can be damaging to the kidneys. Fruits and vegetables high in potassium, such as bananas and avocados, should be avoided if you have renal disease. Furthermore, it is critical to avoid processed and packaged juices because they frequently have extra sugars and preservatives that are damaging to the kidneys.

Finally, choosing the appropriate ingredients is a vital element of juicing success. You may make a nutritious and delightful juice that supports kidney health by combining a range of colorful fruits and vegetables, berries, herbs, and spices, and a source of protein. Remember to limit extra sugars and avoid items that can affect your kidneys.

Incorporating juicing into a balanced diet.

Incorporating juicing into a well-balanced diet is essential for juicing success and kidney health. While juicing has numerous health benefits, it should not be used in place of other nutritious items in your diet. Here are some suggestions for incorporating juicing into a healthy diet:

1. Use Juicing as a Supplement: Juicing can be a terrific method to supplement your diet with extra nutrients, but it should not be used in place of full fruits and vegetables. Juicing should be used as an addition to your usual diet rather than as a replacement.

2. Balance Your Juice with Other Foods: In addition to juicing, consume a well-balanced diet rich in whole fruits and vegetables, lean protein, and whole grains. This will help guarantee that you are getting all of the nutrients your body needs.

3. Restrict Juice Consumption: While juicing can be an excellent way to supplement your diet with additional nutrients, it is critical to limit your juice consumption. Drinking a lot of juice can lead to weight gain and an overabundance of sugar, both of which are bad for your kidneys.

4. Use Nutritious Ingredients: When juicing, select ingredients that are both nutritious and low in sugar. Incorporate leafy greens like kale and spinach, as well as low-sugar fruits like berries, into your juice preparations.

5. Avoid processed juices: Many processed and packaged juices have additional sugars, preservatives, and other potentially hazardous chemicals that might affect the kidneys. To

Juicing for Kidney Health

maintain your kidney health, avoid these sorts of juices and instead produce your own fresh juice at home.

6. Hydrate: It is critical to stay hydrated when juicing. Drink plenty of water throughout the day to help flush out toxins and keep your kidneys working correctly.

Incorporating juicing into a well-balanced diet is critical to juicing success and kidney health. Juicing should be used as an addition to your regular diet, balanced with other nutritious foods, and consumed in moderation. By following these guidelines, you can reap the health benefits of juicing while simultaneously protecting your kidneys.

Making juicing a sustainable habit.

Making juicing a routine is critical to achieving juicing success and sustaining renal health. Here are some pointers to help you make juicing a habit:

1.Start small: Making drastic dietary changes all at once can be stressful. Begin slowly and eventually introduce juicing into your regular routine. Make one juice every day at first, then progressively increase the frequency as you gain confidence.

2. Plan Ahead: Schedule your juicing sessions in advance to ensure that you have all of the necessary components on hand. This can help alleviate the tension and irritation that might result from trying to gather ingredients or prepare your drink on the fly.

3. Set Realistic Goals: For your juicing habit, set realistic and attainable goals. For example, you could start by making juice every morning for a week and progressively increase the frequency to twice a day.

4. Keep it Simple: Choose easy-to-make juice recipes that are simple and quick. This will help to keep you motivated and allow you to create juice on a regular basis.

5. Make Juicing a Habit: Include juicing in your everyday routine, such as drinking a juice with breakfast or as an afternoon snack. The more you practice, the more natural it will become and the easier it will be to keep up.

Juicing for Kidney Health

6.Be Prepared: Make sure you have all of the necessary equipment, such as a high-quality juicer, on hand. This will make it easy to create juice on a regular basis and ensure that you can make juice when you need it.

7. Be Positive: Maintain a positive attitude and focus on the health advantages of juicing rather than the labor required to create a juice. Remember that even minor dietary adjustments can have a significant impact on your entire health, including your kidney health.

Making juicing a routine is critical to achieving juicing success and sustaining renal health. By following these guidelines, you may establish a juicing routine that is simple to maintain and provides long-term health advantages for your kidneys.

Celebrating Progress.

Celebrating milestones and achievements.

Celebrating accomplishments and milestones is a vital aspect of remaining motivated and tracking progress toward kidney health through juicing. This is why:

1. Increases Confidence: Celebrating milestones and achievements increases your confidence and supports the idea that you are progressing toward your goals. This can provide you with the desire and drive you need to keep going on your trip.

2. Increases Motivation: Recognizing and applauding your accomplishments can help you stay motivated and on track. It provides a sense of success and satisfaction, which might assist you in remaining focused and motivated.

3. Achieving a goal, no matter how minor, can bring a sense of satisfaction and pride. Celebrating these accomplishments might make you feel better about yourself and increase your self-esteem.

4. Promotes Positive Habits: Celebrating accomplishments promotes the formation of positive habits and emphasizes the necessity of making positive changes in your life. It also emphasizes the necessity of leading a healthy lifestyle and sticking to your goals.

Juicing for Kidney Health

5. Raise Awareness: Celebrating milestones and achievements raises awareness of your progress and the positive influence your efforts are having on your health. This can help you stay motivated and focused on your objectives.

6. Reinforces Dedication: Celebrating your accomplishments strengthens your commitment to your goals and helps you stay on track. It aids in the formation of a positive behavioral pattern and supports the notion that you are capable of making great changes in your life.

Sharing your accomplishments and milestones with friends, family, or a support group can provide you with a sense of community and shared experience. This can help strengthen relationships and provide encouragement and support.

There are numerous methods to commemorate your accomplishments and milestones, including:

1. keeping a log of your accomplishments

2. sharing your accomplishments with friends and family

3.Indulge yourself with a special treat.

4. Participating in a group or communal celebration

5. Publicly recognizing your accomplishments.

Celebrating accomplishments and milestones is a vital aspect of remaining motivated and tracking progress toward kidney health through juicing. You may enhance your confidence, increase motivation, and reinforce your dedication to your goals by acknowledging and celebrating your accomplishments.

Sharing experiences and successes with others.

Celebrating advancements in kidney health by exchanging knowledge and achievements with others can be quite effective. We can encourage and support others who are going through similar difficulties by sharing our stories, which will make them feel less isolated on their journey. Furthermore, by letting others know what is possible, we might inspire them to keep moving forward on their own journeys toward greater kidney health.

Juicing for Kidney Health

One of the most important advantages of sharing achievements and failures with others is that it can foster a sense of support and community. We demonstrate our concern for others' well-being and foster a sense of connectedness in them when we share our triumphs and experiences with them. People with kidney illness may feel alone and detached from those who do not understand their situation, so this might be extremely crucial for them.

Sharing accomplishments and failures with others can also help put things in perspective, which is another advantage. We open a window into our lives and show others what is possible when we share our experiences and accomplishments. This might provide those who are having trouble with their kidneys' health hope and motivation, which can be extremely useful. One can demonstrate to others that progress can be made even in the face of a chronic ailment by sharing, for instance, how they were able to improve their kidney function through lifestyle adjustments.

Sharing our triumphs and experiences with one another can be good for our own wellbeing. We can better comprehend our personal path and the advancements we have made by thinking back on our experiences and sharing them with others. This may help us feel more accomplished and more confident, both of which may encourage us to keep improving our kidney health.

In the end, communication with others is a powerful method to celebrate advancements in kidney health. We can assist and inspire others and show them what is possible through interacting with others and sharing our experiences. We may all gain from the sense of camaraderie and support that comes from sharing our tales, whether we are listening to others' experiences or discussing our own.

Continuing to set and achieve new goals.

Setting and achieving new objectives for kidney health is a great way to mark accomplishments and keep up the pace of improving one's general well-being. By establishing goals, we may direct our efforts and create a strategy for reaching the desired results. When we achieve our objectives, this can give us a sense of direction and purpose, as well as a sense of accomplishment.

The ability to track our progress is one of the main advantages of creating goals. When we set goals, we have something specific to strive for, and as we move closer to our goals, we can

Juicing for Kidney Health

gauge our success. When we see the results of our efforts, we can maintain our motivation and focus, as well as feel a sense of pride and satisfaction.

Setting objectives also keeps us motivated and focused on maintaining good health. When we have a specific goal in mind, we are more inclined to take steps to achieve it and are more likely to give our health the priority it deserves in our daily lives. This can keep us motivated even in the face of setbacks or other roadblocks by giving us a sense of purpose and direction.

By recognizing accomplishments along the way, setting objectives may also be a way to celebrate progress. For instance, if someone sets a goal to enhance kidney function, they might acknowledge each modest accomplishment they make in that direction, such as cutting back on salt intake or drinking more water. Even before the ultimate goal is reached, this can provide the person with a sense of accomplishment, keep them motivated, and help them gain momentum.

It's crucial to regularly evaluate your progress and make changes as necessary. This can help to maintain the individual's interest and motivation and can help to guarantee that they are moving closer to their goal. If someone sets a goal to enhance kidney function, for instance, they may need to change it if they discover that they are not progressing as quickly as they had planned. The person can continue to celebrate their accomplishment and keep moving toward their goal by constantly reflecting on progress and making modifications as necessary.

The best method to recognize advancement in kidney health is to keep setting and achieving new objectives. We may stay motivated and engaged while assessing our progress toward better kidney health by creating goals and regularly reflecting on our results. Setting and attaining new objectives helps keep us motivated and focused on our journey to improved health, whether we are working toward them alone or with the help of others.

Recap of the importance of staying motivated and celebrating progress in achieving kidney health through juicing.

Maintaining motivation and acknowledging accomplishments are essential steps in juicing for kidney health. As juicing gives the body a concentrated amount of nutrients and antioxidants that can assist in improving kidney function and lowering the risk of renal disease, it can be a very

Juicing for Kidney Health

effective strategy to support kidney health. Juicing has many advantages, but to get the most out of them, you need to stay motivated, keep on task, and recognize your accomplishments.

Improved kidney function is one of the main advantages of juicing. Juicing can enhance kidney health and lower the risk of renal disease by giving the body a concentrated amount of nutrients. For instance, juicing can give the body a lot of antioxidants, which can shield the kidneys from harm and enhance their general performance. Juicing can also aid in reducing inflammation, which is a common contributor to the onset of kidney disease.

Maintaining motivation and acknowledging accomplishments are crucial steps in juicing for kidney health. We are more likely to persist with our juicing routine and get results when we are motivated and laser-focused on our objectives. Setting objectives, monitoring progress, and reminding ourselves of the advantages of juicing for kidney health can help us stay motivated. As an illustration, we could decide to juice a specific number of times per week. We could then keep track of our progress by journaling or by utilizing a monitoring app.

It helps you maintain kidney health by encouraging you to celebrate your accomplishments. We may maintain our inspiration and motivation by acknowledging our accomplishments and the effort we have put into enhancing our health. For instance, we can rejoice whenever we achieve a tiny victory, like juicing for the first time or juicing more frequently. By telling others about our experiences and acknowledging the constructive improvements we have made in our lives, we may also celebrate our progress.

Finally, when juicing for kidney health, it's crucial to be consistent and patient. Despite the fact that juicing can be a highly effective technique to improve kidney health, it is not a quick fix, and results may not be apparent right away. However, by maintaining motivation and acknowledging accomplishments along the way, we can stay motivated and inspired and reach our objective of improved kidney health.

It has been shown to support kidney health and lower the risk of renal disease in a very effective way. We may maximize the advantages of juicing and get greater kidney health by remaining motivated, enjoying achievement, remaining consistent, and being patient. Whether we are juicing for the first time or trying to improve our health, remaining motivated and recognizing

Juicing for Kidney Health

our successes are essential steps toward reaching our objectives and raising our general wellbeing.

Final thoughts on the benefits of incorporating juicing into a healthy lifestyle.

The body and mind can gain a variety of advantages from juicing when it is included in a healthy lifestyle. Incorporating more fruits and vegetables into the diet, which are crucial for optimum health and wellness, may be done quickly and deliciously by juicing. Here are a few more reasons to incorporate juicing into your healthy lifestyle:

Increasing the intake of fruits and vegetables, which are abundant in vitamins, minerals, and antioxidants, is a great way to enhance nutrient intake. These nutrients can aid in immune system support, inflammation reduction, and general well-being. They are crucial for sustaining excellent health.

Supports Weight Management: Juicing is a low-calorie technique to increase nutrient intake; therefore, it can also support weight management. A glass of fresh juice can be substituted for a high-calorie snack to help cut calories and aid in weight loss.

Enhances Digestion: By giving the body nutrients and fiber that are easily absorbed by the body, juicing can help enhance digestion. Juice consumption can aid in removing waste and toxins from the body, enhancing digestion, and avoiding constipation.

Increases Energy and Clarity: Fresh juice contains nutrients that can increase energy and clarity. A rapid energy boost from a glass of fresh juice can aid with concentration, focus, and general mental performance.

Supports Detoxification: By giving the body the nutrients and antioxidants it needs to clean the liver and other organs, juicing can also support detoxification. Fresh juice can aid in the body's detoxification process, improving general wellness and health.

A quick and tasty method to improve health and wellbeing is to incorporate juicing into a healthy lifestyle. Juicing may be a great supplement to a healthy lifestyle, whether you're trying to

Juicing for Kidney Health

increase your nutrient consumption, promote weight loss, or just enjoy a tasty and refreshing drink.

It can have a variety of positive effects on the body and psyche. Juicing can be an important component of a healthy and balanced lifestyle, whether your goal is to enhance your health or you simply want to enjoy a delicious and nourishing beverage. So take full advantage of this fantastic instrument and begin reaping the rewards of juicing right away.

www.ingramcontent.com/pod-product-compliance
Lightning Source LLC
Chambersburg PA
CBHW051552250726
48653CB00004BA/1108